Incorporating Psychotherapeutic Concepts and Interventions Within Medicine

T0134079

This book provides doctors with insights into psychological and relational dynamics to better understand themselves and their patients, deepen their understanding of somatic and psychic dimensions of illness, and give them diagnostic and therapeutic tools to design better treatment procedures for patients.

In the first part of the book, the authors explore cognitive, emotional, and somatic strategies that are supportive of doctors' well-being. In the second part, they introduce theoretical knowledge and applicable skills from psychotherapy that can illuminate the complexity of the doctor-patient relationship, broaden doctors' approaches, and upgrade their communicative skills. The third part introduces some of the basic tenets of somatic psychotherapy that can deepen doctors' understanding of symptoms and illness, providing them with richer therapeutic tools and a deeper knowledge of bodily and psychological aspects, interweaving in a variety of medical conditions.

This text not only provides a helping hand to both doctors and psychotherapists in designing an amalgamated approach to clinical treatment but also provides doctors with better tools for understanding and managing the intricacies of the doctor-patient relationship.

Shamit Kadosh, MD, is a family physician and practicing psychotherapist. She is currently a lecturer at Bar Ilan University (Medicine) and the Shiluv Institute (Psychotherapy). She headed a training program for the residents in family medicine in the Department of Family Medicine in North Israel.

Asaf Rolef Ben-Shahar, PhD, is a psychotherapist, author, and trainer. He founded a number of psychotherapy programs in Israel and the UK. He is the author of four books and numerous papers about psychotherapy. Asaf was editor-in-chief of *The International Body Psychotherapy Journal.*

Incorporating Psychotherapeutic Concepts and Interventions Within Medicine

With the Heart in Mind

By Shamit Kadosh and Asaf Rolef Ben-Shahar

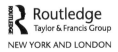

NEW YORK AND LONDON

First published 2020
by Routledge
52 Vanderbilt Avenue, New York, NY 10017

and by Routledge
2 Park Square, Milton Park, Abingdon, Oxon, OX14 4RN

Routledge is an imprint of the Taylor & Francis Group, an informa business

Library of Congress Cataloging-in-Publication Data
A catalog record for this title has been requested

ISBN: 978-1-138-55118-3 (hbk)
ISBN: 978-1-138-55119-0 (pbk)
ISBN: 978-1-315-14751-2 (ebk)

Typeset in Times New Roman
by Apex CoVantage, LLC

In memory of Moshe Shpiler

For his courage, loving kindness, and the inspiration he was for those coping with chronic illnesses

Contents

Introduction

Being a doctor has been a dream for me since my childhood as a daughter to a chronically ill father. I admired doctors; looking up to them, as a little girl, they were like Gods to me. Standing up with their white coats and a serious expression on their face; operating peculiar instruments; and always knowing the answers. Time and again they did their miracles and saved my father's life.

Years have passed; I have become a family doctor. The divine appearance has been cracked; uncertainty and the limits of medical science have been striking to me. Practicing medicine confronted me with a wide breadth of duties and challenges. I was required to endure stressful workloads, manage critically ill patients, make influential decisions under pressure, and encounter human suffering. I was expected to do all that empathically and professionally. It is not surprising, therefore, that like many doctors I found myself stressed, dissatisfied, and sometimes feeling not qualified enough in dealing with suffering of my patients, the complexity of the doctor-patient relationship, communicative intricacies, and psychosomatic symptoms.

Facing these challenges and difficulties, I started my training as a psychotherapist hoping that psychotherapeutic knowledge and experience could be integrated in my clinical practice. After years of training, trying to integrate psychotherapy and medicine into practice and teaching students and residents I have finally started feeling that both disciplines can contribute each other and be applicable in clinical practice contributing to both doctors and patients.

There are two fundamental aspects of medical care. The first is the expert knowledge of diagnosis and treatment; the second is the doctor-patient relationship. Both are necessary for therapeutic goals to be achieved. In the last few decades medical care saw advances in many fields, tremendously affecting those two elements. The recognisable importance of doctor-patient communication and the development of patient-centred approach on one hand, and the accumulating knowledge in psychoneuroimmunoendocrinology and psychosomatic medicine on the other hand, challenge the doctor-patient encounter. This shift in medicine requires doctors to develop new relational skills and therapeutic ones, which are oftentimes missing in their training. The growing gap affects those two fundamental aspects and leads to frustration and helplessness faced by doctors.

This book aspires to introduce and integrate psychotherapeutic knowledge into medical practice, in a way that can be digested, assimilated, and practiced by doctors without attempting to become psychotherapists. Notwithstanding the value of specialised training, the book will provide doctors with better tools for understanding and managing the intricate doctor-patient encounter.

The book is comprised of three parts, each supporting the development of sensitivities, diagnostic tools, and interventional skills which lead to better and more cooperative doctor-patient relationships.

1. Part one: The doctor as a human being, incorporating a doctor-centred approach.

Doctors are confronted on daily basis with human suffering, loss, grief, death, anger, helplessness, accusations, and failures. Coping strategies developed by doctors have received far less study. Trying to protect themselves from being overwhelmed by feelings and the ever-present potential for making a fatal error leads to dissociation, distraction, paternalism, rationalism, self-sacrifice, and self-flagellation. While those strategies may be useful at times, there are substantial costs leading to emotional distress, depression, dissatisfaction, burnout, and somatic symptoms. We wish to support doctors not only in becoming better doctors, but also in cultivating a happier and less distressed professional life.

In this book we explore cognitive, emotional, and somatic strategies to support doctors' well-being. We believe that when doctors work without experiencing high levels of distress, they have greater liberty to think clearly and practice more confidently: in other words, a happier doctor makes for a better doctor.

2. Part two: The doctor-patient relationship, exercising therapeutic skills without being a psychotherapist.

The powerful influence of the doctor-patient relationship on the process and outcomes of care is well recognised and documented. The medical literature is abundant with knowledge about communicative skills. Notwithstanding, creating rapport with patients is far more complex than carrying out communicative skills. Patients arrive at our clinics suffering and anxious, which brings the most primal of human feelings—anger, expectation, blame, helplessness, depression, and (possibly more than anything) fear. It is very difficult not to take this personally. We believe that introducing theoretical knowledge and applicable skills from the field of psychotherapy into medical care can significantly broaden doctors' approach and upgrade their communicative skills. Bringing awareness to the dynamic of transference between doctors and patients, as well as to other psychological phenomena such as self-states, resonance, and projective-identification could illuminate this complex relationship and the mutual influence on each other and better equip the doctor in dealing with highly emotional presentations. Communicative skills such as reflection, empathy, and dyadic regulation will be more achievable facilitating better outcomes of the doctor-patient encounter.

3. Part three: With the body in mind—Incorporating body-mind skills in medical treatment.

Based on accumulating data and research the connection between mind and body and the interface between them is well known. However, so far the medical training has provided doctors with very little satisfactory diagnostic and therapeutic tools for approaching this developing stance. This growing gap leaves the doctors behind with bewildering feelings and frustration with their incapability to provide better health care for their patients. The last part of the book would introduce some of the basic tenets of body psychotherapy knowledge which could deepen doctors' understanding of symptoms and illness, providing them with richer therapeutic tools. Acquaintance with the language of the body, embodied diagnostic tools, the somatic and psychic dimensions of symptoms and diseases is paramount for a deeper and broader understanding of bodily and psychological aspects interweaving in a variety of medical conditions.

The purpose of this book is to introduce doctors with an integrative approach based on theory and clinical experience emanating from two fields—western medicine and body psychotherapy. We do not pretend to train doctors as psychotherapists, but instead to provide them with an applicable therapeutic orientation. Ideally, this book would accompany a similar training program. Psychological and psychotherapeutic understanding could enrich and improve the doctor-patient relationship, as well as contribute to a happier and more satisfied practitioner, a doctor whose practice is closer to the hopes and fantasies he or she had when deciding to train as a doctor.

Part I

The Doctor as a Human Being, Incorporating a Doctor-Centred Approach

1 The Price of Caring

It is the end of an arduous day in the clinic. I am an hour beyond schedule and still need to get over with paperwork before going home, when the nurse is telling me there is one more patient to see. I feel exhausted. I have been taking care of patients all day. I can still feel inside myself Jenifer's anger at me for not helping her with her fibromyalgia pain; Dan's anguished eyes after telling him that cancer is back; my helplessness with Barbara's worsening heart failure and Michael's unexplainable weight loss.

While being flooded by those feelings, I sense myself becoming numb and caring less. I find myself encountering the symptoms and signs instead of the human beings, getting easily angry and impatient while listening to my patients' stories. I try to fight for threads of humanity that I know exist inside, but from time to time they slip away.

What has happened to me? Is this what I was dreaming of?

Being a doctor has awarded me with precious, touching, and fulfilling moments that fill me with gratification and gratitude. Special experiences of intimacy and human care, eureka moments when making the right diagnosis, and times when I feel being attentive and helpful interweave together and keep reminding me of what I appreciate in practicing medicine. Nonetheless, there are times when feelings of helplessness, frustration, and exhaustion take over, fading my expertise and making me care less.

I was a six-year-old child when my professional training as a doctor began. My father's struggle with cancer made me an expert in attending to suffering and alleviating it. It was then when I decided to dedicate myself to medicine. I was inspired by doctors' knowledge and humanity and admired them for saving my father's life time and again. I made a commitment that expertise, humanity, and honesty will be my Northern Star as a doctor, and I promised myself never to forget.

And here I am at the end of the day with my painful familiar feelings of helplessness, anger, and numbness and the remnants of my shattered old dream.

1.1 The Shattered Dream

Practicing medicine confronts us with a wide breadth of duties and challenges. We are required to endure stressful workloads, manage critically ill patients, make influential decisions under pressure, and encounter human suffering. We are expected to do all that empathically and professionally. It is not surprising, therefore, that many doctors may suffer psychological stress and dissatisfaction (Gunasingam et al., 2015). While medical literature is abundant with studies regarding patients' feelings and emotions during the medical encounter, physicians' emotions and their emotional responses have received far less attention (Roter & Hall, 2006). We all want to be empathic, attentive, and lenient with our patients. While being unaware of our emotional responses or trying to supress them (Roter & Hall, 2006), constant exposure to human suffering, demanding patients, and intense levels of stressful work expose us to intensities of feelings and sensations and may predispose us to long-term damages (Hadad & Rolef Ben-Shahar, 2012).

The healthcare field is becoming increasingly aware of the profound impact exposure to human suffering and patients' traumatic stories have on health care providers. Most of us enter the medical profession with strong ideals, beliefs, and faith in our ability to make a difference. As our beliefs become eroded, we might feel disappointed and hopeless (Benson & Margaith, 2005). Our professional lives have become but a faded version of what our dreams once used to be.

Medical training based on scientific objectivity, expertise, and perfectionism that is deficient in an empathic and non-judgemental attitude towards its students and residents, and does not encourage self-compassion and self-care as basic skills, could have significant implications on doctors' coping styles. Facing human suffering and highly demanding duties in such a context might force doctors to survive rather than be fully present.

Is it too much to wish to thrive as doctors?

The following sections explore some research from adjacent fields of care, illustrating the price we pay for our profession of choice, and highlighting some possible directions for reducing the physician's difficulties.

1.2 Vicarious Traumatisation

The concept of vicarious traumatisation (Mac Ian & Pearlman, 1990) describes professional counsellors' complex traumatic reactions deriving from cumulative exposure to traumatic patients. By recognising that trauma may not only expose those directly impacted by it, but might also gravely impact those who come in contact with the trauma sufferer, vicarious traumatisation represents changes in the counsellors' life following working with traumatic material. The reported psychological symptoms attributed to vicarious trauma may include depression, despair, cynicism, and other psychological and physical symptoms (Pearlman & Saakvitne, 1995).

While broadly studied in mental health practitioners, vicarious traumatisation has received very limited attention in medical literature (Palm et al., 2004).

Because encountering human suffering, traumatic, and life-threatening events in people's life is part and parcel of practicing medicine, we believe that vicarious traumatisation has significant implications on doctors and deserves appropriate attention. Studies report high prevalence of doctors feeling emotionally exhausted and stressed, showing diminished interest in their work and experiencing features of burnout (Gunasingam et al., 2015).

1.3 Empathy and Compassion Fatigue

Empathy and compassion have been shown to be an indispensable element in maintaining an effective therapeutic alliance with patients, in delivering high-quality care and increasing doctors' well-being (Gleichgerrcht & Decety, 2014; Neumann et al., 2008).

Empathy is the basis for human connection. It informs us about the other's need and enables us to translate our humanity and act compassionately (Hadad & Rolef Ben-Shahar, 2012). Physician's empathy is defined as the ability of the physician to understand the patient's situation, perspective, and feelings, communicate that understanding and check its accuracy, and act on that understanding with the patient in a helpful way (Mercer & Reynolds, 2002).

Unfortunately, studies illustrate that maintaining appropriate levels of clinical empathy is challenging and empathy declines even during medical school and residency (Neumann et al., 2011; Gleichgerrcht & Decety, 2014).

Why would such an important feature of human interaction be harmed by the practice of medicine?

In describing the phenomenon of empathy fatigue, Stebnicki (2008) believes that it results from a state of psychological, emotional, mental, physical, spiritual, and occupational exhaustion that occurs as the healthcare providers' own wounds are incessantly revisited by their patients' life stories of chronic illness, disability, trauma, grief, and loss. Empathy fatigue may be experienced as an obscure sense of loss, grief, or stress. It has both acute and cumulative emotional, physical, and systemic reactions that are unique to each individual, resulting in varying degrees of professional impairment and competency.

Compassion involves feelings of caring and kindness towards oneself and others in the face of personal suffering combined with the recognition to one's suffering. We may consider compassion as consisting of three fundamental components. First, is the ability to extend kindness to oneself rather than criticise and judge. Second, is the capacity to see human experiences as part of larger humanity rather than as separating and isolating, that is to recognise that our suffering is not unique and singular. The third element refers to holding one's painful thoughts and feelings in balanced awareness rather than over-identifying with them (Neff, 2003, p. 224; Birnie et al., 2010).

Epstein (2017) identifies three components of compassion: noticing another's suffering, resonating with their suffering in some way, and then acting on behalf of another person. He delineates how compassion nourishes the practitioner by releasing endogenous opioids, dopamine and oxytocin which attenuate our own pain, promote a sense of reward, and generate feelings of caring, affiliation, and belonging. Epstein (ibid.) believes that while compassion fills doctors with a deep sense of purpose and well-being, it may also provoke distress and a natural human tendency of withdrawal as a means of self-protection. Sometimes feeling empathetic when there is so much suffering around us can simply prove too much to bear.

Compassion fatigue has been referred to as the emotional 'cost of caring' for others. It is understood as a stress response emerging suddenly as a consequence of working with people who have experienced stressful events. Possible symptoms include helplessness, confusion, isolation, exhaustion, and dysfunction (Figley, 1995; Rudolph et al., 1997).

Medical professionals are continuously exposed to overwhelming situations. Physicians require a facilitative safe-enough environment which could foster connection with empathy and compassion for their patients as well as for themselves.

Unfortunately, when insufficiently attended to, empathy and compassion fatigue may lead to burnout (Benson & Margaith, 2005; Solcum-Gori et al., 2011).

1.4 Burnout

Burnout could be understood as physical, emotional, and mental exhaustion caused by long-term involvement in emotionally demanding situations (Figley, 1995). Burnout is often expressed as a negative shift in the way professionals view people they serve and how they feel about themselves. It encompasses three dimensions: emotional exhaustion, depersonalisation, and reduced personal accomplishment (Gunasingam et al., 2015; Maslach, 2003). Characteristic symptoms include fatigue, exhaustion, inability to concentrate, depression, anxiety, and irritability. The hallmark of burnout is a loss of interest in one's work or personal life (Gundersen, 2001).

Burnout is endemic in healthcare professionals with up to 60% of practicing physicians reporting relevant symptoms. It is associated with various physical problems, substance abuse, higher prevalence of doctor suicide, adverse impact on personal relationships, and lower quality of care (Gundersen, 2001; Irving & Dobkin, 2009; Krasner et al., 2009).

Various causes for burnout have been identified in the literature. Long working hours, poor work-life balance, diminished self-care, denial of emotions and own needs, increased administrative duties, and a perception of loss of control have all been associated with burnout (Gundersen, 2001; Gunasingam et al., 2015; Krasner et al., 2009). All these factors are commonplace in the life of a physician.

Avoiding the temptation to protect ourselves from loss and pain by denial or repression is a difficult practice, particularly since it is almost counterintuitive to allow pain to penetrate us. Remen (2000, 2006) portrays how protecting ourselves from loss by denial rather than grieving our losses is one of the major causes of burnout. She enlightens the significance of grief, self-care, and support in coping with feelings of detachment and burnout. Consider the following case material, the price it takes and the promises it holds:

The nurse opens the door, walking Sara into the room. Her thin, brittle, tenuous body and her pale skin almost hide her warm, vital eyes. She can hardly walk; her lymphoma cells keep spreading in her body despite chemotherapy. I miss her former visits a year ago, coming blissfully with her granddaughter asking me to read letters for her since she couldn't read. It was way before her persisting cough, the mediastinal lymphoma, and chemotherapy.

Her blood count is deteriorating and she is slowly being defeated by cancer.

"You look tired, doctor", she surprises me.

"Just a busy day". I smile at her.

"How are you, Sara?" I ask.

"Well, you know . . . I've known better days. Fever again . . . you know, hospital, antibiotics and so on . . . the regular routine".

I look at her brown, beautiful eyes; sadness is spreading throughout my body when I see her exuberant humanity, slowly giving way to signs of impending death.

"Chemo is not working, ha?" she says.

"I am so sorry", I say and we are holding hands sharing agony together for a few inconsolable yet precious moments reviving my own humanity and compassion.

"Thank you doctor, for everything" she says on her way out, "and take care of yourself".

The door is closed now; it's late at the end of a busy day. I gather my things and go out. I am on my way home to meet my own family. While I can still feel the remnants of the busy day in my body, I can breathe and feel alive. My heart is open again. Sara has helped me renovate the sense of humanity, life, and gratitude in me.

I never saw her again; Sara had died a week later.

We believe that in spite of doctors' cumulative exposure to trauma, stress, and suffering and its impact on their well- being, at the end of the day doctors require self-care strategies that will enable them to continue practicing medicine competently with a sense of meaningfulness and satisfaction engaging them with their original dream. Moreover, we believe this is actually possible.

In the next chapters we will elaborate those issues and introduce our novel notion of the doctor-centred medical care, both theoretically and practically.

Something to Think About:

What makes you feel grateful and fortunate as a doctor?
To what extent do you cherish those precious values?
How close is your practice to your dream?

References

Benson, J., & Margaith, K. (2005). Compassion fatigue and burnout: The role of Balint groups. *Australian Family Physician, 34*(6), 497–498.

Birnie, K., Speca, M., & Carlson, L.E. (2010). Exploring self-compassion and empathy in the context of Mindfulness-Based Stress Reduction (MBSR). *Stress and Health, 26*, 359–371.

Epstein, R. (2017). *Attending: Medicine, mindfulness and humanity*. New York, NY: Scribner.

Figley, C. (1995). Compassion fatigue: Toward a new understanding of the costs of caring. In B. Stamm (Ed.), *Secondary traumatic stress: Self-care issues for clinicians, researchers, and educators*. Lutherville, MD: Sidran Press.

Gleichgerrcht, E., & Decety, J. (2014). The relationship between different facets of empathy, pain perception and compassion fatigue among physicians. *Frontiers in Behavioral Neuroscience, 8*(243), 1–9.

Gunasingam, N., Burns, K., Edwards, J., Dinh, M., & Walton, M. (2015). Reducing stress and burnout in junior doctors: The impact of debriefing sessions. *Postgraduate Medicine Journal, 91*, 182–187.

Gundersen, L. (2001). Physician burnout. *Annals of Internal Medicine, 135*(2), 145–148.

Hadad, E., & Rolef Ben-Shahar, A. (2012). The things we're taking home with us: Understanding therapist's self-care in trauma work. *International Journal of Psychotherapy, 16*(1), 50–61.

Irving, J.A., & Dobkin, P.L. (2009). Cultivating mindfulness in health care professionals: A review of empirical studies of Mindfulness-Based Stress Reduction (MBSR). *Complementary Therapies in Clinical Practice, 15*(2), 61–66.

Krasner, M.S., Epstein, R.M., Beckman, H., Suchman, A.L., Chapman, B., Mooney, C.J., & Quil, T.E. (2009). Association of an educational program, in mindful communication with burnout, empathy, and attitudes among primary care physicians. *Journal of American Medical Association, 302*(12), 1284–1293.

Mac Ian, P.S., & Pearlman, L.A. (1990). Vicarious traumatization: A framework for understanding the psychological effects of working with victims. *Journal of Traumatic Stress, 3*, 131–149.

Maslach, C. (2003). *Burnout: The cost of caring*. Malor Books: Cambridge, MA.

Mercer, S.W., & Reynolds, W.J. (2002). Empathy and quality of care. *British Journal of General Practice, 52*(supplement), S9–S13.

Neff, K.K. (2003). The development and validation of a scale to measure self-compassion. *Self and Identity, 2*, 223–250.

Neumann, M., Edelhauser, F., Tauschek, D., Fischer, M.R., Wirtz, M., Woopen, C., Scheffer, C. (2011). Empathy decline and its reasons: A systematic review of studies with medical students and residents. *Academic Medicine, 86*(8), 996–1004.

Neumann, M., Wirtz, M., Bollschweiler, E., Warm, M., Wolf, J., & Pfaff, H. (2008). Psychometric evaluation of the German version of the "Consultation and Relational Empathy" (CARE) measure at the example of cancer patients. *Psychosomatic Medical Psychology, 58*, 5–15.

Palm, K.M., Polusny, M.A., & Follette, M.V. (2004). Vicarious traumatization: Potential hazards and interventions for disaster and trauma workers. *Prehospital and Disaster Medicine, 1991*, 73–78.

Pearlman, L.A., & Saakvitne, K.W. (1995). Treating therapists with vicarious traumatization and secondary traumatic stress disorder. In *Trauma and the therapist: Countertransference and vicarious traumatization in psychotherapy and incest survivors* (pp. 150–168). New York, NY: W.W. Norton & Co.

Remen, R.N. (2000). *My grandfather's blessings: Stories of strength, refuge and belonging*. New York, NY: Penguin Group.

Remen, R.N. (2006). *Kitchen table wisdom: Stories that heal*. New York, NY: Penguin Group.

Roter, D.L., & Hall, J.A. (2006). *Doctors talking with patients/patients talking with doctors: Improving communication in medical visits*. Westport, CT: Praeger Publishers.

Rudolph, J.M., Stamm, B.H., & Stamm, H.E. (1997, November). *Compassion fatigue: A concern for mental health policy, providers, and administration*. Poster session at the 13th Annual Meeting of the International Society for Traumatic Stress Studies, Montreal, Canada.

Solcum-Gori, S., Hemsworth, D., Chan, W.W.Y., Carson, A., & Kazanjian, A. (2011). Understanding compassion satisfaction, compassion fatigue and burnout: A survey of the hospice palliative care workforce. *Palliative Medicine, 27*(2), 172–178.

Stebnicki, M.A. (2008). *Healing the mind, body, and spirit of professional counselors*. New York, NY: Springer Publishing Company.

2 Fighting for Your Life

John's body is shivering, his shoulders are tightened, and he is trying to straighten his back, while attempting to tell Lisa that being pregnant might be devastating for her. He is an ambitious, first-year resident, and we are in the middle of a course running a demonstrational encounter of breaking bad news. I can feel his anxiety alongside his efforts to be empathic and fully present, when Lisa does not stop sobbing. After a few seconds, he becomes restless, he keeps moving in his chair when he suddenly says loudly and nervously, "just stop crying, calm down".

John falls silent; he is a little embarrassed. "That's exactly what happens when I see patients", he whispers.

"It's overwhelming", I say and he nods.

After discussing and processing the demonstration with John and the other participants, Hanna expresses her wish to participate in a similar demonstrated situation.

She is sitting with a straight back in front of Lisa telling her the bad news. Hanna is an expert in telling bad news all by the rules. She knows how to perfectly execute every step in the process. She is totally focused in conducting the mission. She keeps describing in detail the laboratory results, their meaning, and the deleterious impact of being pregnant on her health. When Lisa starts crying, she looks at her in an expressionless face and tells her calmly, "I am sorry, but you know there's no need to cry. You can adopt children if you really want to be a mother".

"How do you feel, Hanna?" I ask her.

"I am fine, I think I have done it pretty well", she says.

"What do you feel when you look at Lisa?"

She gets a little confused when she says, "I don't really feel right now; I guess I am sorry for her, but I cannot let myself be involved".

"What do you think would have happened if you let yourself be emotionally involved?" I ask her.

Hanna becomes silent, her face softens, a tender aspect of her humanity is being exposed when she says, "My heart will take over my mind".

2.1 Do We Have a Choice?

Perhaps it is true. Perhaps it is impossible to practice medicine and remain emotionally involved. We do not wish to argue that the only way to practice and to live moves through fully feeling whatever is around us. Certainly, there are times when the ability to dissociate, check out, and function without taking things to heart is a gift. Let us postulate for a moment that indeed, the only way we can protect ourselves as physicians from the abundance of physical and emotional pain we are exposed to on a daily basis is to withdraw our emotional responsiveness, to remain as emotionless and rationale as possible. For most of us, it would mean that we spend the lion's share of our lives without feeling: without feeling pain, but also without experiencing connection, joy, love, softness, vulnerability. If this is the case, we may wish to ask ourselves again—is this a life worth living for me? Is this how I wish to live my life?

As human beings we all wish to feel vitality and pleasure, to be both calm and active, to socially engage and communicate. Neuroscientist Stephen Porges (2003) developed the polyvagal theory out of his experiments with the vagus nerve. He introduced us with his novel term of the *social engagement system*. Porges identified a third type of autonomic nervous system response (in addition to the sympathetic and parasympathetic responses) mediated by the ventral vagal complex, which determined our level of consciousness and wakefulness, and helped us navigate relationships.

Using our social engagement system requires a sense of safety. In non-threatening contexts it regulates the sympathetic nervous system, fosters engagement with the environment, and helps us form beneficent social bonds. When we feel threatened and unsafe, the social engagement system's function is at stake and defence mechanisms arise (Ogden et al., 2006). To reiterate, Porges demonstrates how the ventral vagal complex together with social network systems serve to regulate hyperarousal and stress. Our anxiety regulation is thus both internal (biopsychological) and external (social).

We naturally expend substantial efforts in order to avoid confronting stressful, painful, and devastating emotions. We are blessed with various defensive strategies that allow us to evade intense emotional pain. We tend to develop creative and habitual modes and methods of managing stress and other upsetting emotions. Basic human emotions evoke what psychology identifies as ego defences and coping styles. The difference between defence mechanisms and copying styles rests in conscious agency. Both are ways of dealing with adversity and with psychological disequilibrium, yet while defence mechanisms operate on an unconscious level, coping strategies are considered to be conscious processes (Plutnick, 1989; Cramer & College, 1998). The more we are able to understand our emotional triggers, the more we are able to respond through coping strategies and make conscious decisions about how we navigate our emotional responses.

A defence mechanism is an unconscious psychological mechanism that alters veridical perception and functions to reduce excessive anxiety. This is not a pathological response; we all do it. An adverse reaction to pain is a hallmark of any living organism. Yet while defence mechanisms are an essential part of the normal human mind, they might also result in undesirable consequences depending on the frequency and intensity of their use (Freud, 1936; Loewenstein, 1967). Responding to a physical attack by running away or attacking back could save our lives, responding similarly to arguing with our partner, when the same biological functions are triggered, might not be as useful.

The more common defence mechanisms will be briefly explained below. Becoming familiar with these mechanisms and learning to increase the ability to respond rather than react will facilitate the capacity to make informed choices. This, in turn may not only improve doctor's communication with patients, but also protect the physician's psychological well-being.

As doctors we are obliged to withstand human suffering and attend to highly emotional and stressful situations. We are trained on the foundation of scientific objectification, exalting mental distance as a way to protect us from becoming wounded by our challenging work (Remen, 2006). This is oftentimes confused with resilience. It is therefore only natural that we employ psychological defence mechanisms in order to protect ourselves, even when this entails denying our own emotions and needs. This denial, however, comes at a cost, both professional and personal.

When John and Hanna met Lisa, they were both confronted with a common and highly emotional situation, manifesting different defence mechanisms in order to protect themselves.

Despite their unavoidable commonness and influential impact on doctors' function and well-being, medical literature lacks sufficient papers dealing with doctors' defence mechanisms in the medical encounter.

In this chapter we will delineate common defence mechanisms in healthcare providers, examining their advantages and disadvantages, and embolden individual introspection of your own unique defensive responses in common medical scenarios.

2.2 Common Defence Mechanism in Healthcare Providers: Creative Ways to Refrain From Painful Feelings

Defence mechanisms are not unique to doctors. All humans employ protection as the most nature response to avoiding hurting. Yet, certain professions predispose us to greater and more frequent encounters with pain and, subsequently, to greater activation of these defence mechanisms. As previously mentioned, practicing medicine confronts us with intricate and painful circumstances, which might provoke intense emotions. Throughout medical school, residency, and clinical practice, we are trained to be authoritative, knowledgeable, and self-confident (Epstein, 2017). We learn to disregard, disrespect, and frequently block our own helplessness and emotional soft-spots. Doctors may thus be unaware of their emotional responses; they may suppress them or try to avoid emotionally demanding or arousing situations (Roter & Hall, 2006). These unconscious processes may obliviously arouse defence mechanisms and psychologically detached demeanour.

1. **Dissociation.** Consider this: you have a severe headache. Suddenly you realise there is an interesting programme on the TV. As you watch it, you become absorbed in the programme. The headache is gone, only to return when the programme is over. Dissociation is a socio-biological and psychological phenomenon, whereby part of our experience is detached from the entirety of our experience. Its major characteristic involves a detachment from reality in order to minimise or tolerate stress. Dissociation can be normative and indispensable for survival (e.g., not experiencing severe acute pain), and it can be regarded as a defence mechanism. Many of the defence mechanisms involve a certain level of dissociation (Rolef Ben-Shahar, 2014).

2. **Denial** could be defined as an unconscious refusal to face and accept certain facts and aspects of reality. Insofar as this reality is highly upsetting and threatening, denial can be a very useful defence mechanism (Baumeister et al., 1998; Laplanche & Pontalis, 1973). For some people, refusing to accept their limitations leads to unfathomable success. However, denial could prove fatally dangerous. One example could be a diabetic man who keeps insisting that he is not diabetic, repeatedly endangering himself with his diet. Many doctors, for instance, are in denial of their own basic needs throughout their training and work. On one hand, refraining from being in touch with psychological and physical needs makes it possible to function competently for long hours, but on the other hand doctors pay high prices that impact their health and well-being (Lazarus, 1983).

3. **Repression** is an active pushing down of feelings, the cognitive and emotional effort to ignore or divert attention from threatening stimuli. It is the process of actively and forcibly ejecting threatening material out of the conscious mind (Freud, 1961; Weinberger & Davidson, 1994). When a patient provokes in me uncomfortable feelings, I might try to avoid it by attempting to forestall it from entering consciousness. While breaking the bad news to Lisa, Hanna is repressing her painful feelings towards her. Unlike denial, which is a refusal to recognise an aspect of our experience, repression is a forced pressing down of an experience or memory.

4. **Suppression**, as compared to repression, refers to a conscious decision to delay paying attention to a thought, emotion, or need in order to cope with the present reality. It allows the individual to hold all conflictual and upsetting components in mind and then postpone the action. Suppression, as opposed to repression, makes it possible later to access uncomfortable and distressing emotions. It constitutes a requisite and useful coping strategy. Confronting death and human suffering might waken painful feelings

and memories in me, and occasionally I need to put them aside while working in order to function. I am aware of them and I choose to not engage with them for a while. Hopefully, I will have the opportunity to process these feelings later on.

5. **Projection** refers to attributing one's own traits to other people. It can be seen as a defensive if perceiving the threatening trait in others helps the individual avoid recognising it in himself (Freud, 1961). By attributing one's own unacknowledged and unacceptable thoughts or emotions to another and allowing their expression, it reduces anxiety. When I feel guilty for not succeeding in managing my patient's diabetes, I might blame her for her partial compliance with her diet and medications instead of being empathic and encouraging. When John demands Lisa to calm down, he projects his overwhelming feelings on her. Sometimes feelings such as anger, helplessness, or guilt towards our patients are too troubling to admit, and we attribute those feelings to originate from them.

6. **Distraction.** Look, a bird . . . Distraction is a means of deciding to put off thinking or feeling distressing thoughts or emotions by temporarily focusing our attention towards something less threatening. Using the computer in the medical encounter is a common way of distraction that might enable us to take some time and calm ourselves (as does cigarette smoking).

7. **Intellectualisation** is an unconscious way of isolation that involves a mental gap or barrier between some threatening cognition and other thoughts and feelings (Baumeister et al., 1998). Emotional language is innately different from cognition. One cannot reduce emotions into intellectual argument. It does not stop us from trying, though. When we lose a patient, for example, and feel guilty, we can repeatedly go through the medical procedure and tell ourselves that we have done everything we can, attempting to avoid the pain and guilt by leaning against factual data. Concentrating on the intellectual components of a situation, isolating their emotional meaning, and thinking about them in affectively bland terms, create distance from the associated anxiety provoking emotions. When Hanna lengthily describes Lisa her blood tests results and rushes into finding solutions such as adopting a child, she intellectualises the highly emotional situation so she will not have to attend the overwhelming feelings.

8. **Objectification** in the medical encounter is the process of scrutinising the disease element as separate from self. As doctors we are trained to define the disease scientifically by physio-chemical measures and refrain from thinking about the human experience of being ill. By objectifying a patient we deal with the illness, the organ, or the symptom instead of with the person. This is far easier, as illnesses or symptoms have no feelings, expectations, and disappointments. Objectification protects us from confronting ourselves as sufferers and dying human beings (Tauber, 1999). Treating the pneumonia in room nine or the diabetic with haemoglobin A1C 9 are common examples of this phenomenon. Gupta (2011) honestly shares with us in his paper how his entire world centred on "veins", so much that

he unconsciously categorised his patients as either having "good veins" or "difficult veins". It is important to note that mostly there is no malicious intent in objectification.

9. **Altruism and self-sacrifice.** What would Jesus do? Saving fantasies of grandeur that manifest in abandoning our own feelings and needs to attend to another person are most common interlocked psychological strategies among healthcare providers. Altruism is a means of transforming uncomfortable feelings and thoughts by serving others. Doctors tend to make significant personal sacrifices for their patients, often sacrificing personal time, sleep, hobbies, and family time in order to satisfy their patients and meet their needs. While being constructive it may result in self-sacrifice of own basic needs. When not balanced, it may have adverse effects on doctors' well-being. Chronic altruism refutes our true limitations and boundaries, and moreover colludes with a fantasy of being more-than-human, someone who can live without what most people need.

2.3 The Prize and the Price

Defence mechanisms may result in healthy and unhealthy consequences depending on the circumstances, frequency, and intensity with which they are being applied. While we have been trained to be scientific, objective, and emotionally self-controlled in order to be considered competent doctors, we are also unrealistically expected to be empathic, compassionate, and immersed in suffering daily without being touched. Our humanity, which makes it possible for us to execute our professionalism in a helpful way, also carries another side of exposing us to pain, suffering, and adversity.

Emotional distance protects us from becoming wounded by this challenging work. Without underrating the benefits, we cannot ignore the price we pay for being distant and emotionally detached.

Tauber (1999) describes science as providing a veil for life-and-death experiences that are immediately and profoundly presented to the doctor by the seriously ill. Remen (2006) elaborates the issue by displaying how detachment and objectivity refrains us from our own human strengths. She proclaims that emotional distance makes us far more vulnerable than compassion and simple humanity. It disconnects us from being alive and fully experiencing the whole variety of feelings.

Throughout the courses we run, we ask participants to share some of their most fulfilling moments as doctors. Most of them disclose that human moments of intimacy and compassion are of paramount value for them. When distancing from our humanity, we lose one of the most valuable awards of our profession.

Furthermore, denial and repression of our feelings and needs have an adverse impact on our well-being and health. Excessive inhibition of emotional self-disclosure is also associated with negative interpersonal, psychological, and health consequences (Larson & Chastain, 1990).

Gleichgerrcht and Decety (2014) demonstrate how professional experience seems to desensitise physicians to the pain of others without necessarily helping them down-regulate their own personal stress. Pain perception might affect the levels of empathy physicians feel towards their patients. They assume that minimum levels of empathy are necessary to benefit from positive aspects of professional quality-of-life in medicine.

Concurrent with the effects on our well-being, psychological distant behaviours might be painful for our patients and have unfavourable effect on the medical encounter (Amir & Kalemkerian, 2003).

Based on our professional and personal experience, we premise that cultivating self-care and self-soothing strategies along with fostering more adaptive and beneficent coping styles can enable doctors be touched and emotionally connected and become more satisfied and grateful. We need our social engagement system to reside in our daily practice as doctors, so as to have latitude to choose our responses more freely, socially engage, and communicate with our patients empathically. Expecting doctors to be compassionate, empathic, and fully present in the face of suffering and highly emotional load without providing them with strategies advocating their well-being is like trying to build the second floor in the absence of the first one.

In the next chapters we will discuss the value of grief; we will explore healthier coping styles and introduce you with various ways of self-care and self-soothing.

Something to Think About

> Identifying your common defence mechanism and cultivating self-awareness is an essential component for engaging with healthier coping styles.
> What are your commonly used defence mechanisms?
> How do you tend to respond to common scenarios (demanding patient, breaking bad news, attending human suffering, etc.) in your practice?
> When do you tend to feel emotionally disconnected?
> When do you feel connected to your emotions and humanity?
> To what extent are you in touch with your basic needs?

References

Amir, M., & Kalemkerian, G.P. (2003). The art of oncology: When the tumor is not the target run for your life: The reaction of some professionals to person with cancer. *Journal of Clinical Oncology, 21*(19), 3696–3699.

Baumeister, R.F., Dale, K., & Sommer, K.L. (1998). Freudian defense mechanisms and empirical findings in modern social psychology: Reaction formation, projection, displacement, undoing, isolation, sublimation, and denial. *Journal of Personality, 66*(6), 1081–1124.

Cramer, P., & College, W. (1998). Coping and defense mechanisms: What's the difference? *Journal of Personality, 66*, 6.

Epstein, R.E. (2017). *Attending: Medicine, mindfulness and humanity*. New York, NY: Scribner.

Freud, A. (1936). *The ego and the mechanisms of defense*. New York, NY: Hogarth Press.

Freud, S. (1961). Repression. In J. Strachey (Ed. and Trans.), *The standard edition of the complete works of Sigmund Freud* (Vol. 14, pp. 143–160). London: Hogarth Press. (Original work published in 1915).

Gleichgerrcht, E., & Decety, J. (2014). The relationship between different facets of empathy, pain perception and compassion fatigue among physicians. *Frontiers in Behavioral Neuroscience, 8*(243), 1–9.

Gupta, P. (2011). Humanity in medicine. *Journal of Medical Ethics and History in Medicine, 4*(3).

Laplanche, J., & Pontalis, J-B. (1973). *The language of psycho-analysis* (D. Nicholson-Smith, Trans.). New York, NY: W.W. Norton & Co.

Larson, D.G., & Chastain, R.L. (1990). Self concealment: Conceptualization measured and health implications. *Journal of Social and Clinical Psychology, 9*(4), 439–455.

Lazarus, R.S. (1983). The costs and benefits of denial. In S. Breznitz (Ed.), *The denial of stress*. New York, NY: International Universities Press.

Lowenstein, R.M. (1967). Defensive organization and autonomous ego functions. *Journal of the American Psychoanalytic Association, 15*, 795–809.

Ogden, P., Minton, K., & Pain, C. (2006). *Trauma and the body: A sensorimotor approach to psychotherapy*. New York, NY: W.W. Norton & Co.

Plutnick, R. (1989). Measuring emotions and their derivatives. In R. Plutnick & H. Kellerman (Eds.), *The measurement of emotions* (pp. 1–35). San Diego, CA: Academic Press.

Porges, S.W. (2003). Social engagement and attachment: A phylogenetic perspective. *Annals New York Academies of Sciences, 1008*, 31–47.

Remen, R.N. (2006). *Kitchen table wisdom: Stories that heal*. New York, NY: Penguin Group.

Rolef Ben-Shahar, A. (2014). *Touching the relational edge: Body psychotherapy*. London: Karnac Books.

Roter, D.L., & Hall, J.A. (2006). *Doctors talking with patients/ patients talking with doctors: Improving communication in medical visits*. Westport, CT: Praeger Publishers.

Shanafelt, T., Adjei, A., & Meyskens, F.L. (2003). When your favorite patient relapses: Physician grief and well-being in the practice of oncology. *Journal of Clinical Oncology, 21*(13), 2616–2619.

Tauber, A.I. (1999). *Confessions of a medicine man: An essay in popular philosophy*. Cambridge, MA: Massachusetts Institute of Technology Press.

Weinberger, D.A., & Davidson, M.N. (1994). Styles of inhibiting emotional expression: Distinguishing repressive coping from impression management. *Journal of Personality, 62*(4), 587–613.

3 Encountering Suffering

I am walking down the road on my way to his house. Despite the beauty of the flowers and the shining sun, my body is contracted and my breath is heavy when I enter Jeffery's house. He is one of my favourite patients. Whenever he enters the clinic, he fills the room with his blissful and sparkly energy. I miss this Jeffery; the one he used to be before his abdominal pain, the vomiting, and the jaundice. The one before diagnosed with metastatic carcinoma of the pancreas.

He is lying on his couch fighting for each breath. His cachectic body and inflated abdomen fill me with despair and agony. His wife is busy cooking, hoping he might eat something, anything. His daughter is vehemently searching for any new experimental treatments that might help. We focus on pain management, his lack of appetite, and his weight loss. Looking through the window I notice how the flowers' vivid colours highlight Jeffery's signs of death. We are all trying to ignore and avoid mentioning the one and the only word that is screaming in its absence . . . death.

Heavily breathing and feeling dizzy, I suddenly find myself a few years ago next to my father's bed in hospital. He is gasping for each breath, struggling with intolerable pain; death is spreading leaving no cell in his body untouched. Doctors and nurses come and go, take blood tests, measure his temperature and blood pressure, and take care of his hydration. But no one dares to say the word death.

And here I am next to Jeffery, fighting my own breath, trying to regulate my own anxiety.

"You look exhausted, Jeffery", I say." You can hardly breathe". He turns his anguished eyes at me and nods, he can hardly speak. I sit next to him; I gently put my hands on his abdomen, when he takes my hand squeezing it. His eyes are wide open attempting to say something. "You can tell me", I whisper, "I am listening".

His words are fighting their way out, his entire body is vibrating when they finally find their way out and he says decisively, "I want to die in hospice".

The intense silence evolves into painful words and crying when his startled wife and shocked daughter hear his unexpected wish.

Both sorrow and relief fill my heart as I see them arguing, crying, and hugging. They are finally talking honestly and openly about Jeffery's imminent death.

There is no escape; there is no cure. The living organism experiences suffering. From birth, through illness to death, life is imbued with beauty, love, and with pain and suffering. There is no way escaping it.

3.1 Suffering

Suffering is an inevitable aspect of human experience which touches each one of us throughout life. It can be addressed in a myriad of ways and can be given a variety of definitions based on diverse points of view. Each one of us has his own unique view of suffering based on his own biography, personality, education, and culture. Some of us might see suffering as something that might need to be endured, minimised, relieved, explored for meaning or may even give rise to growth (Cuttcliffe et al., 2015).

Suffering manifests in numerable guises: stress, depression, interpersonal conflict, confusion, and despair. It may be existential, such as sickness, old age, and dying or it might have a more personal flavour.

Doctors encounter human suffering on a daily basis and yet medical literature pays little attention to suffering (Cuttcliffe et al., 2015)

Epstein (2017) defined suffering as a personal and pervasive distress affecting someone's identity. Cassell (1982) was one of the pioneers to initiate a serious discussion regarding the nature of suffering in medicine. He recognised three aspects of suffering. The first involved the whole person and required a rejection of the historic dualism of mind and body. The second referred to a threat to the intactness of oneself causing significant distress. Regarding the third aspect, Cassell stressed how suffering could occur in relation to any aspect of life. He highlighted psychological, existential, social, financial, and spiritual domains of suffering other than the disease or disability itself.

To reiterate, suffering is an individual experience for each person—it is not the adverse stimuli but instead the response to it, the subjective experience. Hence, similar events may cause different levels of distress and suffering for each individual. For a forty-year-old businessman, travelling all over the world, the recent diagnosis of diabetes mellitus may endanger his functioning and cause much suffering, while for a sixty-year-old woman, who have been devoted to taking care of her children for years, it might be perceived as an opportunity for self-care.

As doctors we have to address various dimensions of suffering in order to fully accompany our patients. The subjective, rather than objectified and measurable aspects of suffering make dealing with it a human, rather than a scientific act. While the enormous significance for patients is well known, many doctors find this kind of involvement challenging, too painful, time consuming, and sometimes impossible to implement.

Moreover, attending to suffering requires tuning in to one's own pain and suffering, which is not an easy choice. As human beings we prefer happy and healthy people. Alas, these rarely show up at our clinics. Intimate emotional relationships with disabled, diseased, and dying individuals forces us to face our own vulnerability, fears, helplessness, and mortality

(Amir & Kalemkerian, 2003). On one hand, Tauber (1999) explicated that young medical students were generally poorly equipped emotionally to cope with the demanding responsibility of treating severely ill patients. He emphasised that they had little intimate experience of attending to and witnessing pain and death. On the other hand, some of the people attracted to medicine are the ones who are familiar with their own suffering or their relatives'. We believe that previous experience with suffering does not necessarily protect us and may even predispose us to overwhelm and emotional distress. At the same time, when unprepared, doctors will resolve to implementing strong defence mechanisms against suffering.

As thoroughly detailed in the previous chapter, our painful feelings in the face of suffering may provoke a variety of defence mechanisms leading to avoidance of recognising and addressing our patients' suffering. In their unique touching and honest way, Amir and Kalemkerian (2003) awarded us with a glimpse to Amir's own experience as a patient coping with cancer. They depicted a variety of distancing strategies used when facing with the stress of interacting with a diseased individual. They noted how people might be ignorant of suffering and refrain from asking the patient how he or she felt. They also mentioned various possible reactions to the patient's sadness and other painful feelings suggesting that these feelings were not perceived as legitimate or acceptable.

When I met Jeffery in his unbearable suffering and impending death, I was overwhelmed by his agony and by my own unprocessed loss. Trapped in my emotional overflow, I refrained from talking with him about his feelings and his death and I struggled to attend to his experience.

Tauber (1999) illustrated how clinical language reinforced doctors to distance from the suffering patients. He exemplified doctors' tendency to not speak of the person, but of the case (or similarly to speak directly to a patient's relative rather than to the patient themselves), reminding us that we are trained to look for facts and objective information and tend to avoid seeking the subjective experience of the sufferer.

While having the potential of rewarding our patients and us as doctors, fully attending to our patients' suffering obliges us to open our hearts; be in touch with our fears, helplessness, and losses; and grieve. This is by no means an easy task, and sometimes not fully possible. But it is a rewarding effort. We believe that doctors need to cultivate their own resources, self-care, and coping strategies so they can be there without endangering their well-being. This, of course, requires maturity.

3.2 Grief

Grief is a response to a significant loss, which is associated with suffering of variable duration. It is grounded in and manifesting through our psychoneurobiological system. Mourning is the shared expression of a grief experience. Together, grief and mourning constitute the grief process, representing movement from life through death and back into life again (Bruce 2002, 2007).

There are numerous offered models describing and defining the grief process. In *On Death and Dying,* Elisabeth Kübler-Ross (1969), a psychiatrist and thanatologist, published her seminal five steps model of grief process. Based on her observations she described a five-step paradigm which included: denial, anger, bargaining, depression, and acceptance. She perceived the process of grieving as a progressive one, while at times these stages were overlapping or coexisting. She considered the completion of this five-stage process as necessary to allow for a healthy return-to-life.

Recent models of grief process (Bowlby, 1980; Parkes, 1988) add to Kübler-Ross's model by highlighting an element of shock and disbelief as an expression to a shutdown, caused by a distressful situation needed for self-protection. They also mention components of disorganisation, despair, and depression as a phase on the way towards healing. Those models are not always linear but could recycle through recollection, or some triggering experience. They all point to the irrational, all-consuming subjective experience of grief.

If grieving process is arrested at some point, the grief experience might become intensified, remain fixated, or incomplete.

The grief process calls for both inwardly experiencing and outwardly expressing the reality of loss through mourning; it demands us to tolerate pain while caring for ourselves, to relate the experience of loss to context of meaning, and to develop an enduring support system that can provide us with a strengthening brace while healing takes place (Worden, 1982).

Emotions during grief are functional and useful guides. They hold something important for us to learn in this process, and should not be perceived as dysfunctional conditions to be extinguished or overcome (Neimeyer, 2001). Emotions are compasses which guide us through the grieving process into a recovery and adaptive everyday life.

3.3 Doctors' Grief

Can we sincerely experience so much loss without being touched and impacted?

While physicians are expected to be honest, compassionate, and professional guides who are capable of advising and comforting patients and their families in most devastating times, we are just as human as our patients. We encounter unbearable moments with our patients, forge close relationships with many patients, and share intimate moments of sorrow and triumphs, pain, and hope (Shanafelt, Adjei, & Meyskens, 2003). There is no doubt that patients, families, and healthcare providers share some of the same needs when confronted by loss and suffering. They need time to feel, understand, and process their losses. They need to grieve. Unfortunately, doctors commonly have little time to process their own sorrow about their patients' suffering and loss (Meier, 2001), and they lack appropriate conditions that might enable the process. In effect, doctors are left to bear the results of accumulated incomplete grief processes. Attempting to deal with grief solely through intellectual and defensive means further exposes physicians to stress and adverse physical and psychological symptoms.

In their study, Granek and his colleagues (2012) explored and identified oncologists' grief over patient loss and the ways in which this grief might have affected their personal and professional lives. They found that oncologists struggled to manage their feelings of grief along with the detachment they felt necessary in order to competently manage their caseload. Most commonly reported feelings were those of failure, self-doubt, sadness, powerlessness, and guilt. The study indicated that grief in the medical context was considered shameful and unprofessional. Even though participants struggled with feelings of grief, they hid them from others, since expressing such emotions was perceived as a sign of weakness. The participants noted that their unacknowledged grief led to inattentiveness, irritability, emotional distress, and burnout. These are all common symptoms of incomplete grief (Bowlby, 1980; Kübler-Ross, 1969). Half of the participants pointed out that their discomfort with their grief over patient loss affected their treatment decisions, their ability to communicate about end-of-life issues with patients and their families, and made them distance and withdraw from patients. The authors (Granek et al., 2012) viewed their participants' grief as smoke. They depicted it as intangible, invisible yet pervasive and sticking to physicians' clothes when they went home after work. They suggested that doctors' failure to deal appropriately with grief from patient loss may negatively affect both physicians and patients.

3.4 Processing Suffering: First, Be Human, No More, No Less

Processing and attending suffering are intricate and complex issues. We do not pretend to have magic solutions or a to-do list for coping with vulnerability, uncertainty, tidal waves of helplessness and guilt, treatment failures, medical futility, loss, and death. Nevertheless, we would like to share with you some of our experience with regards to attending and processing suffering, hoping each one of you would find his own unique way of beneficent coping.

Interestingly, the first 'noble truth' in Buddhism is the existence of suffering: an acknowledgment that there is suffering in this world. The basic principle of Buddhist doctrine aim is to help raise our understanding above the level of automatic response into the realm of transformation. The first noble truth refers to suffering as unavoidable. Although as doctors much of our effort works to obscure this truth (or fight against it, forever in vain, with all our might), an important first step is to accept this notion. When a suffering patient comes to us, we do not always have the capacity to remove the suffering. Yet, we know that isolation, objectification, and diagnostic labelling may increase suffering and should be minimised. Especially in suffering, we can deeply join one another in our common vulnerability. It is the acceptance of this simple truth of suffering that is, as we understand it, at the core of healing.

Being aware of the inability to bring up end-of-life issues with Jeffery was an important first step which led to an awareness of feelings of helplessness, fear, and sorrow. Cultivating self-awareness of our feelings and our perception of suffering is an essential first step. We all hold different perceptions regarding suffering and our duties as physicians. When encountering suffering and death some will tend to build walls for protection, some will blame themselves or others, and others will feel most comfortable trying to fix things. Being mindful to our perceptions, feelings, and reactions enables us to choose another way of handling the situation. Epstein (2017) explicates how doctors feel most comfortable fixing things. He demonstrates how a diagnose-and-treat approach might avert doctors' attention from the full range of their patients' suffering. If we hold (consciously or unconsciously) such an approach we are prone to feel guilt, failure, and helplessness—since suffering does not go away. Being aware and mindful might help us take another perspective. Accompanying and being present with our diseased and dying patients has an ineffable potential in relieving their unbearable suffering. When we broaden our duty beyond curing, we can appreciate the profound significance of our human presence in alleviating our patients' suffering.

Human beings are meaning-seeking organisms (Frankl, 1956), and our ability to attribute meaning to our experiences greatly influences the course of emotional healing or symptomatology. The way we perceive suffering has a profound impact on how we process it. It has been recognised since ancient times that the experience of suffering can give rise to growth. One of the most famous quotes of Rumi, the Sufi poet, says that the wound is the place where the light enters you. Holding this kind of view means seeing suffering as an inevitable aspect of the human condition with a potential of making meaning. We believe that rethinking our views of suffering, and considering how they might help us and our patients discover meaning in experience might be helpful.

Cassell (1982) argued that exploring the meaning of suffering could affect the severity and quality of a person's distress and the sense he made of it. Victor Frankl (1973) in his book *The Doctor and the Soul* wrote of the importance of finding meaning in suffering. After greatly suffering in a concentration camp during World War II, he concluded that almost any suffering can be tolerated if it can be imbued with meaning. He developed a form of psychotherapy (Logotherapy) dedicated to the discovery and creation of meaning within our life, and our suffering. Remen (2000) emphasised the importance of acceptance and meaning. She asserted that attending to suffering started with the realisation that our loss has become part of us and has changed our lives in such a profound way that it was impossible to go back to the way things used to be before. She assumed that something in us could transform suffering into wisdom. Remen described the process of letting feelings of anger, blame, and the sense of injustice go, until being left with a deeper sense of value in life and a greater capacity to live it.

Failure to accept limitations may result in feelings of guilt and helplessness. While we are committed to our patients, we may feel personally responsible for our inability to produce miracles. Despite our best intentions and efforts, we often lack the capability to reverse the course of diseases. Accepting this painful fact allows us to be present, alleviate our intense feelings, and pursue the meaningful work of helping patients accept their illnesses and make significant decisions concerning their lives.

Self-acceptance of our humanity, incapability, feelings, and reactions is of paramount importance. We are in the front of the most unbearable human conditions trying to do our best. Alongside our skilful expertise in diagnosing, treating, and being empathic and compassionate, we also make mistakes, find ourselves impatient and detached from time to time. While trying to cultivate a compassionate and empathic approach towards our patients, we have to develop this kind of attitude towards us.

Another important issue is making space for us to grieve like everyone else. As previously depicted, we acknowledge the profound importance of grieving and the price of withholding from the process. Adequate personal time to grieve our own losses can bring healing and prevent struggles at work from spilling over into personal relationships (Meier et al., 2001). As mentioned before doctors tend to conceal their painful emotions, feeling it is inappropriate to express their feelings and share. Regular meetings with colleagues to share grief, mistakes, and suffering as well as rewards of medicine can strengthen self-awareness, alleviate loneliness, promote a sense of connection, reaffirm professional values' elucidating existential aspects of practicing medicine, and enrich practice (Shanafelt et al., 2003).

Of a paramount importance is strengthening our inner resources, cultivating self-care strategies and pursuing ways of nourishment. We will elaborate this issue in the following chapters.

While confronting daily with suffering is challenging, we hope each one would find his own way of coping in a compassionate manner, fostering his own well-being. We will have moments of feeling open-hearted, flickering of epiphany and a sense of gratitude and fulfilment alongside of moments of despair, detachment, and loneliness. Even while writing these lines we can feel how we fluctuate between the intention to write from the depth of our vulnerable open-hearted human experience to the force pulling us towards psychological distance and intellectualisation of one of the most powerful, intense, unavoidable, and painful human experience.

The sun set and twilight fell in the end of another busy day in the clinic. I am walking down the road on my way to his house again. Despite the darkness, I can still imbibe the beautiful sight of the flowers. Sadness is expanding in me; I am on my way to see him for the last time. Tomorrow morning, he will leave his home to die in another bed, in another place, in hospice.

He is lying on his couch fighting for each breath with his cachectic and exhausted body. His beautiful brown eyes calm me with their serenity. His eyes blink in agreement when I approach him and quietly ask permission to give him a hug. My arms are around his gaunt and tired body. Precious moments of our ten-year relationship fill me with warmth and open my heart wider. "Goodbye, Jeffery", I whisper with tears in my eyes. A small tear down his cheek and his grateful eyes are answering me goodbye.

Something to Think About

How do you deal with ending in your personal life?

What role models do you have for humanly and professionally dealing with endings?

What would happen if you allowed yourself to be touched in face of grief?

References

Amir, M., & Kalemkerian, G.P. (2003). Run for your life: The reaction of some professionals to a person with cancer. *Journal of Clinical Oncology, 21*(19), 3696–3699.

Bowlby, J. (1980). *Attachment and loss: Loss, sadness and depression* (Vol. 3). New York, NY: Basic Books.

Bruce, C.A. (2002). The grief process for patient, family, and physician. *Journal of Osteopathic Association*, 102, S28–S32.

Bruce, C.A. (2007). Helping patients, families, caregivers, and physicians, in grieving process. *Journal of Osteopathic Association, 107*, ES33-ES40.

Cassell, E.J. (1982). The nature of suffering and the goals of medicine. *New England Journal of Medicine, 306*(11), 639–645.

Cuttcliffe, J.R., Hummelvol, J.K., Granerud, A., & Eriksson, B.G. (2015). Mental Health nurses responding to suffering in 21st century occidental world: Accompanying people in their search of meaning. *Archives of Psychiatric Nursing, 29*(1), 19–35.

Epstein, E. (2017). *Attending: Medicine, mindfulness and humanity*. New York, NY: Scribner.

Frankl, V.E. (1956). From psychotherapy to logotherapy. *Pastoral Psychology, 7*, 56–60.

Frankl, V.E. (1973). *The doctor and the soul: From psychotherapy to logotherapy*. New York, NY: Vintage Books.

Granek, L., Tozer, R., Mazzotta, P., Ramjaun, A., & Krzyzanowska, M. (2012). Nature and impact of grief over patient loss on oncologists' personal and professional lives. *Archives of Internal Medicine, 172*(12), 964–966.

Kübler-Ross, E. (1969). *On death and dying*. New York, NY: Macmillan.

Meier, D.E., Back, A.L., & Morrison, R.S. (2001). The inner life of physicians and care of the seriously ill. *Journal of American Medical Association, 286*, 3007–3014.

Neimeyer, R.A. (2001). *Meaning reconstruction and the reality of loss*. Washington, DC: American Psychological Association.

Parkes, C.M. (1998). *Bereavement: Studies of grief in adult life* (3rd ed.). Madison, CT: International Universities Press.

Remen, R.N. (2000). *My grandfather's blessings: Stories of strength, refuge and belonging*. New York, NY: Penguin Group.

Shanafelt, T., Adjei, A., & Meyskens, F.L. (2003). When your favorite patient relapses: Physician grief and well-being in practice of oncology. *Journal of Clinical Oncology, 21*(13), 2616–2619.

Tauber, A.I. (1999). *Confessions of a medicine man: An essay in popular philosophy*. Cambridge, MA: Massachusetts Institute of Technology Press.

Worden, J.W. (1982). *Grief counseling and grief therapy: A handbook for the mental health practitioner*. New York, NY: Springer Publishing Company.

4 The Doctor-Centred Medical Care

Rachel is a well-experienced family physician who has just shared with us her difficulties with her demanding patient Mike. We are in the middle of a course dealing with the challenges of the doctor-patient communication, when Rachel is recreating an intricate situation in a role-play with one of the participants.

Her breath is shallow and fast, her shoulders tightened, and she is trying her best to be polite and empathic while facing his demand for an urgent CT scan for his tension headaches. She listens to him carefully, making an effort to engage with his agenda and addressing his fears while explaining to him there is no necessity for a CT scan. Her body shrinks and her lips quiver when Mike gets angry at her.

"I cannot do it", she suddenly stops the role play. "It's not fair. I have to be empathic, compassionate, and professional and to always think about the well-being of the patient". Her eyes are wide open with vital anger when she says, "What about me? How can I be empathic and attentive to my patients, when I am exhausted? I am so busy providing patients the best of my skills, implementing the patient-centred medicine principles that I have no time to eat drink or breathe. I am really asking you, what about me?"

Her emotionally laden words strike the silence in the room. Her body softens; tears are in her eyes when she looks at us. Rachel dares to honestly raise our unspoken frustration and arouse important thoughts and conflicts concerning the tension between the well-being of patients and that of doctors.

What if? What if we dare to follow Rachel's distressed question and join her in asking 'What about us?' What would happen if alongside the patient-centred principles we will also tune-in to our own needs and well-being? Could this be a genuine possibility?

Bodhisattva is a Buddhist pledge to seek enlightenment in order to help others reach enlightenment too. It is an oath of committing to oneself in recognition that before we can truly help others, we need to be attentive to where we are. It is an oath of leading by example. As parents we already know the huge impact that self-care has on our children's well-being. While flying in an airplane we are told to put on our own oxygen mask before we do that for our children. We recognise that attending to our own needs and well-being is not only necessary for us, but also frees us to be better parents, to meet our children's needs with greater patience, compassion, and efficacy.

So how come we are confused, embarrassed, and ashamed of our basic needs as doctors?

The pledge to care for the patient irrespective of any factor and to place him in the focus of our attention is one of the foundations of the medical practice (Tauber, 1999). Nearly all medical schools incorporate some form of professional oath into their graduation's ceremonies. It might be any version of the modern Hippocratic Oath, Maimonides prayer or another version, but they all exalt the principles of being in service for the sick in their distress at any time and at any hour and maintain their deportment while keeping the patients' interests and well-being foremost (Bardes, 2012; Hulkower, 2009).

In this chapter we will discuss the principles of the patient-centred medical care, while presenting our understanding of an old-new notion, the doctor-centred medical care. We will try to integrate those two concepts and to examine feasibility of both in the medical encounter.

4.1 Patient-Centred Medical Care

Patient-centred care is a core value of medicine for many doctors. It had grown alongside the humanistic psychology movement (Rogers, 1951), which recognised the centrality of the patient's subjectivity (patient as a person) for cooperation, and for recovery. While historically medicine practice has been physician centred, we are in the midst of a professional evolution of seeking to focus medical attention on the patient's needs and concerns rather than doctors'. Physicians have begun to incorporate patients' perspectives considering cultural traditions, their personal preferences and values, family situation, and lifestyles (Cliff, 2012; Laine & Davidoff, 1996; Stewart et al., 2000).

Many have contributed to the evolution of this eminent and influential concept. Psychoanalyst Enid Balint (1969) coined the term and suggested a form of mini-psychotherapy that general practitioners could provide patients with psychosomatic aspects in their illness. Engel (1977) proposed the seminal concept of the biopsychosocial model that addresses the patient, his social context in which he lives, and the psychological impact of illness. The profound developing of the doctor-patient relationship understanding and the significant discernment between "disease" and "illness" (Cassel, 1985) has also contributed to the evolution of the patient-centred medicine.

The major components of this approach are exploring various dimensions of the patient's illness experience, addressing and understanding the whole person, finding common ground regarding management with the patient, and enhancing of the patient-doctor relationship (Stewart et al., 2000). Developing the patient-centred approach requires us to focus on doing what's best for our patients and their families, recognising the individual needs of each patient and delivering care in a healing environment that supports our patients' physical, emotional, and spiritual needs (Cliff, 2012).

Research indicates that patient-centred encounters result in better patient satisfaction, higher physician satisfaction, fewer malpractice complaints, improved health status, and increased efficiency of care by reducing diagnostic tests and referrals (Kaplan et al., 1989; Levinson et al., 1997; Roter, 1989; Roter et al., 1997; Stewart et al., 2000).

Then how come it is so challenging and complex?
Let's go back to Rachel's question, "What about me?"

The patient-centred approached developed out of a need to fully recognise the patients as people. It derived from an understanding that people need to feel recognised and seen as people in order to cooperate and relate effectively. The patient-centred approach has done exactly that, yet it had omitted an important factor—the doctor as a person, the physician's subjectivity.

How many of us dare to ask this question at the end of a busy day?

In the previous chapters we have depicted the common and concerning phenomena of doctors' empathy and compassion fatigue and the resulting burnout.

We believe that understanding and interpreting the patient-centred concept as an approach that prioritise the patient's well-being over the doctor's might stake a position that respects, appreciates, and encourages an attitude that addresses doctors' needs and fosters their well-being.

4.2 Doctors' Well-Being

The term *wellness* captures the intricate and multifaceted nature of doctors' physical, emotional, and mental health; it goes beyond the absence of distress and encompasses qualities of fulfilment and thriving (Wallace et al., 2009; Shanafelt & Habermann, 2003).

The acknowledgement of us being human with our own needs creates the ground that can sprout the seeds of our well-being and cultivate them.

The most fundamental needs we all have as human beings are basic physical ones together with the need for human connection and meaning. We also have individual needs influenced by our own physical health and personality (Suchman & Ramamurthy, 2008). In his influential paper, 'A Theory of Human Motivation', Abraham Maslow (1943) illustrated the hierarchy of needs, presented as Maslow's pyramid of needs. He portrayed five layers of needs, with the largest most fundamental ones at the bottom, to psychologic needs in the middle, and fulfilment ones at the top. From the bottom of the hierarchy upwards, the needs are: physical, safety, social, esteem, and self-actualisation. Maslow claimed that needs lower down in the hierarchy must be satisfied before individuals can attend to needs higher up. Notwithstanding the abundance of opportunities for intimate human contact, precious moments of meaning and gratitude our clinical work provides us with, it also makes constant demands jeopardising our own basic needs and well-being.

Research implies that physicians tend to give suboptimum attention to self-wellness (Wallace et al., 2009). They are not good at tending to their needs, they tend to refrain from seeking help from others, they are ignorant and indifferent towards their own health and are used to functioning when unwell (Arnetz, 2001; Firth-Cozens, 2001; Pullen et al., 1995; Taub et al., 2006; Thompson et al., 2001). Doctors are prone to lose sight of the balance between their own enrichment and depletion. They usually become so externally attuned that they lack the capability of being in touch with their own needs and taking care of themselves (Suchman & Ramamurthy, 2008).

Several causes have been attributed to the missing quality of self-care in medical practitioners. Among the most common are a perceived stigma of being incapable of coping associated with seeking help, medical training cultivating unrealistic self-expectations and self-sufficiency, a feeling of pressure from both patients and colleagues to appear physically well as an indicator of medical competence, and professional and organisational barriers contributing to reluctance to discuss health concerns with colleagues (McKevitt & Morgan, 1997; Suchman & Ramamurthy, 2008; Thompson et al., 2001; Wallace et al., 2009).

There is growing evidence alluding to influential detrimental consequences of physicians' lack of self-care on the individual and the health care system. Increasing awareness of the importance of physician wellness will probably lead to increased doctors' satisfaction and overall well-being and would reduce likelihood of distress and burnout (Coster & Schweble, 1997; Roter & Hall, 2006; Wallace et al., 2009). While until recent years scant attention was directed towards preventive measures of burnout among doctors, there has been growing interest and development of attunement aimed at fostering wellness and applying necessary self-care skills for clinicians (Irving et al., 2009; Taub et al., 2006; Weiner et al., 2001).

"I am so disappointed in myself", Rachel shares her feelings with us.

"I know what I am supposed to do, but I feel exhausted, angry and distressed that I have to fake it".

She keeps talking anxiously about her eroding confidence as a doctor, and her immense frustration confronting demanding patients like Mike.

"I used to like being a doctor, I think I still do, but it feels as if nobody notices all my efforts and attempts, I can barely find time to drink water while working, I am totally immersed with my patients, and then comes a patient like Mike and I lose it".

Her shallow breath deepens, her tightened muscles soften and the anger spreading her body slowly wanes. She is relieved.

We all share similar feelings. We discuss our basic physical needs as human beings, the need to share, to be seen, and to have boundaries. We remind each other of various resources that we already have summoning them to our space.

Rachel, supported by us and resourced, feels much better.

" Maybe we can give it another try", I suggest Rachel.

"How would it be if you meet Mike again attuned to your own needs and resources? How would it be if you encounter him devoted to your well-being as well as his?"

Silence in the room; her eyes are wide open looking at me befuddled.

"But how can I do that? How can I meet my patient and stay attuned to myself at the same time"?

4.3 Doctor-Centred Medical Care

The beautifully engraved words, 'These are the duties of a physician: First . . . to heal his mind and give help to himself before giving it to anyone else', on the Epitaph of an Athenian Doctor, are in the foundation of the doctor-centred medical care.

How would the Epitaph of an Athenian doctor get along with the Hippocratic Oath?

Bardes (2012), in his enlightening perspective, warns us that addressing the patient-centred medicine as a rhetorical slogan might delude us to a position that perceives other points of view as unethical and forbidden doctor centred. He believes that patients and physicians should meet as equals, exchanging different knowledge, paying attention to their needs and concerns without claiming a position of centrality. He finds the metaphor of a pair of binary stars orbiting a common centre of gravity a much more appropriate one than the metaphor of a Ptolemaic universe revolving around either the physician or the patient.

Implementing a doctor-centred attitude in medicine means valorising, appreciating, and addressing doctors' needs and wellness as prominent qualities. It requires a shift in healthcare perspective to recognise and affirm doctors' physical, emotional, and spiritual needs and the necessity of doctors' self-care. It means a return to relating to ourselves and to our clients as first and foremost human beings.

Humanity can be expressed when we feel safe and nourished.

We all have buds of empathy, compassion, and humanity that wait to be watered so they can burgeon and fully express themselves. When these virtues are regarded as skills to be taught theoretically, we limit their authenticity and quality. The true application of those precious virtues requires a supporting environment and self-care.

We believe that incorporating a doctor-centred attitude is a prerequisite for the patient-centred medicine evolution, and that these could be dialogic and complementary. When we are aware of our needs, connected to our resources and feel nourished, we can deliver better service to our patients based on the principles of the patient-centred stance. Neither the patient-centred practice nor the doctor-centred one can go too far without the other. These are not irreconcilable perceptions, but rather the contrary. Integrating both perspectives nourishes each other and enables a more balanced and human medicine practice to sprout.

> *Rachel takes a deep breath; she is drinking a glass of water, connecting with her inner resources we have just discussed. Although not without feeling guilty, she is hesitantly willing to try being attuned and committed to her needs, resources, and wellness when encountering Mike. Her eyes meet Mike's demanding utterance. He raises his voice, claims a CT scan, and accuses her for malpractice. Rachel's breath gets faster; she loses her upright position and her all body contracts. I stop her for a moment. I ask her to notice her feelings and thoughts.*
> *"I am afraid, I lose my confidence . . ." she whispers.*
> *"What do you need right now in order to feel better?" I ask her.*
> *"Well, I guess I need to remember that I am a good doctor and I know what I do. I also need to remember that his anger is a result of his fear and frustration . . . and I would like to be able to put boundaries".*
> *She takes a few breaths trying to connect with her resources and regulate her feelings. She straightens up in her chair looking at his eyes. No longer ensnared in a whirlpool of overwhelming feelings, aware of her needs and resources, she can be fully present and meet Mike with her empathic assertiveness.*

References

Arnetz, B.B. (2001). Psychosocial challenges facing physicians of today. *Social Science & Medicine, 52*(2), 203–213.

Balint, E. (1969). The possibilities of patient-centered medicine. *The Journal of the Royal College of General Practitioner, 17*(82), 269–276.

Bardes, L. (2012). Defining "patient-centered medicine". *New England Journal of Medicine, 366*, 782–783.

Cassel, G. (1985). *Talking with patients*. Cambridge, MA: Massachusetts Institute of Technology Press.

Cliff, B. (2012). The evolution of patient-centered care. *Journal of Healthcare Management, 57*(2), 86–88.

Coster, J.S., & Schwebel, M. (1997). Well-functioning in professional psychologist. *Professional Psychology: Research and Practice, 28*, 5–13.

Engel, G.L. (1977). The need for a new medical model: A challenge for biomedicine. *Science, 196*, 129–136.

Firth-Cozens, J. (2001). Interventions to improve physicians' well-being and patient care. *Social Science & Medicine, 52*, 215–222.

Hulkower, R. (2009). The history of the hippocratic oath: Outdated, inauthentic, and yet still relevant. *Einstein Journal of Biology and Medicine, 25-26*, 41–44.

Irving, J.A., Dobkin, P.L., & Park, J. (2009). Cultivating mindfulness in health care professionals: A review of empirical studies of Mindfulness-Based Stress Reduction (MBSR). *Complementary Therapies in Clinical Practice, 15*(2), 61–66.

Kaplan, S.H., Greenfield, S., & Ware, J.E. (1989). Assessing the effects of physician-patient interactions on the outcomes of chronic disease. *Journal of Medical Care, 27*(S1), 10–27.

Laine, C., & Davidoff, F. (1996). Patient-centered medicine: A professional evolution. *Journal of American Medical Association, 275*(2), 152–156.

Levinson, W., Roter, D.B., Mullooly, J.B., Dull, V.T., & Frankel, R.M. (1997). The relationship with malpractice claims among primary care physicians and surgeons. *Journal of American Medical Association, 277*, 553–559.

Maslow, A.H. (1943). A theory of human motivation. *Psychological Review, 50*(4), 370–396.

McKevitt, C., & Morgan, M. (1997). Anomalous patients: The experiences of doctors with an illness. *Sociology of Health & Illness, 19*(5), 644–667.

Pullen, D., Lonie, C.E., Lyle, D.M., Cam, D.E., & Doughty, M.V. (1995). Medical care of doctors. *The Medical Journal of Australia, 162*(9), 481–484.

Rogers, C.R. (1951). *Client-centered therapy*. Boston, MA: Houghton Mifflin.

Roter, D. (1989). Which facets of communication have strong effects on outcome: A meta analysis. In M. Stewart & D. Roter (Eds.), *Communicating with medical patients*. Newbury Park, CA: Sage.

Roter, D.L., & Hall, J.A. (2006). *Doctors talking with patients/patients talking with doctors: Improving communication in medical visits*. Westport, CT: Praeger Publishers.

Roter, D.L., Stewart, M., Putnam, S.M., Lipkin, M., Stiles, W., & Inui, T.S. (1997). Communication patterns of primary care physicians. *Journal of American Medical Association, 227*, 350–356.

Shanafelt, T.D., & Habermann, T.M. (2003). The well-being of physicians. *American Journal of Medicine, 114*(6), 513–519.

Stewart, M., Brown, J.B., & Donner, A. et al. (2000). The impact of patient-centered care on outcomes. *Journal of Family Practice, 49*, 796–804.

Suchman, A.L., & Ramamurthy, G. (2008). Practitioner Well-being (pp. 51–56). In M. Feldman & J. Christensen (Eds.), *Behavioral Medicine: A Guide for Clinical Practice*. USA: McGraw-Hill Education.

Taub, S., Morin, K., Goldrich, M.S., Ray, P., & Benjamin, R. (2006). Physician health and wellness. *Occupational Medicine, 56*(2), 77–82.

Tauber, A.I. (1999). *Confessions of a medicine man: An essay in popular philosophy*. Cambridge, MA: Massachusetts Institute of Technology Press.

Thompson, W.T., Cupples, M.E., Sibbett, C.H., Skan, D.I., & Bradley, T. (2001). Challenge of culture, conscience, and contract to general practitioners' care of their own health: Qualitative study. *British Medical Journal, 323*(7315), 728–731.

Wallace, J.E., Lemaire, J.B., & Ghali, W.A. (2009). Physician wellness: A missing quality indicator. *Lancet, 374*(9702), 1714–1721.

Weiner, E.L., Swain, G.R., Wolf, B., & Gottlieb, M. (2001). A qualitative study of physicians' own wellness-promotion practices. *Western Journal of Medicine, 174*, 19–23.

5　Generative Cognitive, Emotional, and Somatic Strategies for Self-Care

Barbara is a dermatologist, who sought psychotherapy for stress management. Upon taking some history, I learn that Barbara works over 60 hours a week, excluding paperwork and admin. She sees her children in the morning and, if lucky, just before bedtime. When I ask her about her last holiday, she laughs at me. After a month I discover that Barbara has only one legitimate way for winding down after a stressful day—alcohol. At the end of a long day, the last thing she wants is to share or speak to anybody. Barbara only noticed that there was a problem when she started experiencing disturbing symptoms at work: her hands were not as stable, she forgot patients' histories, and had a few blackouts. It was only when her husband threatened to leave if she didn't seek help that Barbara called.

Can Barbara survive without drinking? What would happen if we took away her evening winding down habits? She will be left without any down-regulating agent. Psychotherapy proves almost contradictory, at least at first, to her physician's creed: do your best. Somehow, do your best does not self-apply.

How often have you found it difficult to go to work? How burdened do you feel by the needs of your patients? Have you ever wondered how can you make it through each day intact?

In the previous chapters we have depicted the intricacies of practicing medicine, defence mechanisms we inevitably use, and the encumbrance of attending to suffering. We have discussed the epidemic of burnout among doctors and its detrimental implications.

In the last chapter we have introduced you the revisited doctor-centred medical approach and its foundations. In this chapter we wish to elaborate on the applicability of the doctor-centred model by fostering helpful resources and providing you with skills for self-care. We will interweave practices originated from various disciplines and endeavour to make it applicable for clinical use.

A prerequisite for applying the doctor-centred model is to inculcate a sense of permission and faith in the importance of self-care, and to understand and internalise the fact that it is our responsibility to find ways for cultivating our well-being. Nobody will do if for us, and that endeavour would also entails fighting off systemic and administrative pressures to remain completely focused on others. Nurturing well-being is a process requiring work and investment on a regular basis. Furthermore, we have to let go of the common belief that self-care is in opposition to the idea of serving our patients with devotion.

Research implies that learning self-care techniques can affect educational and training experiences of counselling students (Baker, 2003; Weiss, 2004). In a qualitative research examining the impact of providing students with self-care skills and fostering self-awareness, Chambers et al. (2006) show us that the art of self-care has a significant impact on students' personal and professional life.

Epstein (2017) denotes the paramount importance of self-awareness to warning signs, to an honest self-appraisal, and to the importance of cultivating resilience in difficult times. Resilience has been found as a main factor in well-being and inversely related to burnout (Russo et al., 2012; Southwick & Charney, 2012). Epstein (2017) describes three valuable "reminders" (p. 167) regarding resilience. The first refers to the fact that resilience is a capability that we can cultivate with an appropriate training. That is, it is not a trait but a skill. He asserts that doctors can gain more control over their well-being and develop healthier ways to relate to stress. The second reminder is related to his opinion that engaging with difficult situations instead of withdrawing fosters well-being. In his third reminder he highlights the importance of a sense of community in the health care community.

We believe that applying regularly self-care practices, developing and connecting to a variety of resources, and developing mindful self-awareness cultivate well-being and enable the formation of healthier coping strategies. In the next section we will introduce you with practical skills of self-care, a variety of resources to connect to, and further broadening ways to cultivate self-awareness and self-regulation.

5.1 Resources

We are all rewarded with numerous internal and external resources that help us properly maintain our personal and professional life (Ogden & Fisher, 2015). Internal resources refer to personal strengths and competencies developed over time within us, while external ones reside outside us in our environment. There are sundry categories of resources some of which we find of paramount importance in medical care. In this chapter we focus on emotional, cognitive, somatic, and relational resources.

Being aware of our full-range of feelings, expressing and communicating them, self-regulating and tolerating intricate emotions effectively and utilising them to guide action are all emotional resources (ibid.). Knowing oneself is a starting point for later discerning feelings, thoughts, and behaviours which support or hamper our health. This too is a skill rather than a given trait, and as such it commands practice and cultivation. In medical practice we need to be able to reflect on our own feelings and actions, avow our vulnerabilities, and admit our needs (Suchman & Ramamurthy, 2014). When we encounter our so called 'unprofessional' feelings such as frustration, anger, helplessness, deep sorrow, or insecurity arising in us, we can engage with those inevitable feelings, self-regulate, and process them with less overwhelm, withdrawal, or dissociation.

Cognitive resources attribute to our personal philosophy regarding life, belief system, way of thinking, values, and meaning. They have profound impact on the way we perceive suffering and respond to; how we comprehend our roles as doctors and behave; how we imbue meaning and self-compassion to our practice and let ourselves define the framework by which we summon self-care. Throughout life we internalise and develop attitudes, values, and core beliefs stemmed from our families, cultural environment, and life experience. Since these factors filter our perceptions and form our behaviour, we should broaden our awareness so we can decide which parts are resourcing and which ones need to be changed (Suchman & Ramamurthy, 2014).

Our bodies are inextricably linked with our cognitive and emotional realms. Somatic resources include physical actions, capacities, and functions that provide a sense of well-being and competency on somatic level and have the faculty to positively affect how we feel (Ogden & Fisher, 2015). With Barbara, for example, emotional interventions proved only partially useful. Taking a twenty-minute jog every other day, however, completely changed her life. Somatic resources support our well-being and may foster our self-regulatory abilities. Most common practiced somatic resources refer to different kinds of physical activities such as playing sports, dancing, yoga, etc. Less known but highly efficient somatic resources are derived from the field of body psychotherapy. These somatic capacities include somatic awareness to postures, gestures, and senses; breathing techniques; centring and grounding skills. Recognising and deepening our somatic resources will help us self-regulate, regain a sense of being connected with ourselves, and respond more adaptively to adversity with more flexibility.

Relational resources refer to our capabilities of communicating, reaching out to others, setting boundaries, giving and receiving emotional support.

Each one of us has his own unique composition of resources. We propose here that acknowledging our resources, strengthening and reconnecting with them on a regular basis, and addressing them as an integral part of practicing medicine can significantly support our well-being and improve our professional efficacy.

5.2 Mindfulness as a Means of Self-Awareness

Observe, record, tabulate, communicate.
Use your five senses.
Learn to see, learn to hear, learn to feel, learn to smell, and know that by practice alone you can become expert.

William Osler

Each human experience encompasses somatic, emotional, and cognitive aspects. For instance, when I encounter a demanding and furious patient,

I might feel my heart pounding, my breath becoming shallow, and my body leaning back (somatic); I may feel frightened and helpless (emotional); and I might think I am too weak and incapable of setting boundaries (cognitive).

Naturally, we attempt to push inconvenient sensations, emotions, and thoughts away from our awareness, so that we do not have to deal with them. Notwithstanding, we have already shown in the previous chapters that doctors' self-awareness is of paramount importance for both doctors' well-being and patient satisfaction.

Mindfulness can be defined as an awareness of the present experience with acceptance, non-judgement, trust, and curiosity. It is a skill for tuning in to our inner experience, observing and naming the moment-by-moment of each of its component (thoughts, emotions, and sensations) without suppression or avoidance with the aim of helping people be fully present each moment of their lives (Germer, 2005; Kabst-Zinn, 2003; Ogden & Fisher, 2015; Neff, 2003).

Practicing medicine mindfully means we listen to signals coming from our inner being, slow down, and become curious. We direct our attention to our body sensations, our emotions, our thoughts and notions. Step by step, vague sensations and obscure feelings will unfold and shed light on an intricate situation, illuminate our core beliefs, and help us be aware of our needs. With time and practice we will become increasingly familiar with our behavioural patterns, common assumptions we have, and typical coping strategies we use. We will start asking ourselves questions regarding our well-being and basic needs such as: How do I feel now? Am I tired? What do I need now so I can feel better? Our evolving mindful self-awareness will, hopefully, help us deal with overwhelming feelings, promote of self-care and well-being, enhance self-compassion, and decrease personal distress (Birnie et al., 2010; Epstein, 1999; Irving et al., 2009; Krasner et al., 2010).

Consider this common scenario in medical practice while we also attend to our bodily sensations, emotions, and thoughts mindfully.

You have been working for many hours, listening attentively to your patients, examining them, ordering tests, and prescribing medications. You were also called twice for urgent situations to deal with and you are far beyond schedule. You still have a few patients to see before you go home, when your patient comes in angrily. "I have been waiting too long for you", his eyes are burning. "It is always the same . . . I don't understand . . . why does it always have to be like that?" he is looking at you furiously.

Sounds familiar?

We all have to deal with angry patients, but each one of us will react and respond in his unique way and use his own coping strategies. Let us try to practice mindfulness together.

Sit in a quiet place, feel your body touching the chair, your feet touching the floor, and just observe your inner experience.

Notice your breath, is it shallow or deep? Fast or slow?

Notice your posture, how aligned is your upper body? How contracted or relaxed are your muscles?

Notice your body's sensations (heaviness, tightness, tension, impulse for a movement, etc.) Notice your emotions right now (joy, sadness, frustration, etc.) and open your mind to your thoughts and beliefs (Nothing will help; Maybe there is a chance I can feel better, etc.)

Now, try to track a similar memory of yours.

We will begin by exploring body awareness.

Sit quietly, imagine the event and observe your body sensations with curiosity, acceptance, and no judgement, as if you were simply gathering data.

Be mindful to your breath, posture, gestures, and body sensations.

For example, I might feel my chest tightened my breath shallow, the muscles of my upper limbs contracted, my body leaning back, and my back curved forward.

Our body reacts in its own language, communicating through sensations, postures, gestures, movements, and breath. Our sense of self and the way we communicate is affected by our physical reactions and habits (Ogden & Fisher, 2015). When my breath becomes shallow, my chest tightens and my posture is curved forward, it might not only convey implicit meaning of helplessness to my patient, but also to me. Body awareness may help me change the implicit communication I have in this situation by taking a few deep breaths and assume a more aligned posture. This kind of simple intervention might relieve my stress and facilitate in setting boundaries empathically. Moreover, awareness to body sensations may reveal our bodies' basic needs (thirst, hunger, tiredness, etc.) so we can try to fulfil them.

Now, let us move on with mindful emotional awareness.

Go back to your memory and your body sensations and be mindful to your emotions.

Ask yourself how you feel right now. Can you name your feelings and accept them nonjudgmentally? Observe subtle nuances of feeling tones and mood.

For instance, I might feel frightened and attacked alongside feeling helpless and angry.

Doctors respond to patients with myriad of emotions that can affect both the medical care they provide and their own well-being, especially when unexamined and unconscious (Gartrell et al., 1992; McCue, 1982; Pellegrino, 1993; Zinn, 1988). Unexamined emotions such as anger, frustration, sense of failure, helplessness, fear, grief, need to rescue, and desire to avoid patients may all have considerable impact on physicians. Professional loneliness, loss of sense of meaning, cynicism, hopelessness, chronic anger, loss of sense of the patient as a fellow human being, depression, and chronic loss of engagement and satisfaction are amongst the most common consequences of unexamined emotions (Gartrell et al., 1992; McCue, 1982; Novack et al., 1997; Pick, 1985; Yamey & Wilkes, 2001). Meier et al. (2001) describe a model for enhancing doctors' self-awareness, which includes recognising and naming of the feeling, accepting its normalcy, and considering possible connections between emotions and behaviour. They assert that emotions should not be treated as a disorder, but need to be acknowledged and understood.

Emotions tend to have a wavelike quality; an emotion reaches a peak and fades. By avoiding an intense emotion, we hinder the normal decline of our emotions' intensity. When I am aware of and nonjudgmentally present with my fear, sense of helplessness, and anger encountering my patient, I facilitate the process of self-regulation and I have more choices regarding my behaviour. Practicing mindfulness cultivates our capacity to observe, monitor, and modulate our own emotional reactivity. Instead of blaming ourselves or others, becoming overinvolved or dissociated when faced with complex emotional situations, we could instead observe our reactions and make better choices that will enhance quality of care and our well-being (Epstein, 2014). Mindfulness helps us free ourselves from passively reacting to our emotional experience, and become active agents in structuring our responses.

Another aspect of our human experience encompasses our thoughts.

Let us go back to the previously mentioned scenario and mindfully attune to our cognitions. Be aware of your thoughts, interpretations, meanings, and beliefs about yourself and about your patient.

For example, I might notice having thoughts like "It is my fault" and "Nobody can see how hard I have been working".

Cognitions are thoughts describing our experience by conveying interpretations, meanings, and theories. They may become generalised into unrecognised erroneous beliefs, which play a large play in perpetuating our feelings about ourselves and our patients (Ogden & Fisher, 2015). We are all trapped in our habitual thinking-patterns and captured by our belief system. Exposing thinking habits such as shame, criticism, self-flagellation, and unworthiness are of paramount importance. When I am aware of my thoughts of self-blame and dissatisfaction, I can observe these adverse thoughts and be less identified with them and, therefore, less caught up and swept away by aversive reactions. Moreover, the ability to recognise and be in touch with my needs to be seen and listened to, can direct me to seek for the support I need.

Being mindful to our own personal needs is of great importance. It can significantly ameliorate our own well-being by helping us be in touch and attuned to our needs and by motivating us to seek the support we need and the resources we have to connect with.

Exercise: Practicing Mindfulness

Mindfulness is a skill that can be developed through practice. This exercise is recommended as a regular practice to improve your mindfulness skills.

Sit comfortably and allow your eyes to gently close if it feels right.

Take a few moments to feel your body, and the sensations associated with touch in the places you are in contact with the floor.

Let your attention settle on your breath, feel the rising and falling of your chest and abdomen.

Observe your posture, how aligned is your back?

Be aware of your body sensations like racing heart, butterflies in your stomach, vitality, tightness, heaviness, tiredness, hunger, thirst, etc. Simply take note of these without attempting to change any of your sensations.

Be aware of your emotions: fear, sadness, anger, disappointment, help-lessness, joy, etc. Observe subtle nuances of feelings and mood.

Focus on the qualities of your thoughts. Observe how thoughts arise and pass away. Note their content and their emotional charge.

If possible, continue with that for a few minutes with patience, accept-ance, and no judgement.

Now go to consider a complex situation with a patient.

Let yourself be present in the situations.

Use your senses to be present in those moments: see the sights, hear the voices, smell the odour.

Let your attention settle on your body, feelings, and thoughts with acceptance as described above.

5.3 Self-Compassion

Self-compassion is an active cultivation of kindness and caring towards oneself in the face of personal inadequacies, mistakes, failures, painful life situations, and suffering. Kindness, a sense of common humanity, and mindfulness are fundamental elements of self-compassion (Neff, 2003). It encompasses three essential components: (1) self-kindness and understanding toward ourselves rather than judgement and self-criticism; (2) perceiving our own experiences as part of humanity rather than as separating and isolating; and (3) being mind-fully aware of painful thoughts and feelings rather than over-identifying with them (Neff, 2003). To reiterate, self-compassion involves a kind and balanced approach to oneself—not too tight, not too loose.

Growing research indicates that self-compassion is associated with decreased psychopathology, more moderate reactions, increased resilience, and numer-ous psychological strengths, enhanced motivation, and improved interpersonal functioning (Bernard & Curry, 2011; Heffernan et al., 2010; Leary et al., 2007; Neff et al., 2007).

Being self-compassionate in medical practice means neither refraining from painful experiences nor over-identifying with them. Rather, it means being pre-sent and responding kindly with the intention of resolving rather than blaming, shaming, or self-flagellation (mostly masked by the need to be right). It involves a gentle and encouraging inner conversation, acknowledging our problems and shortcomings, our pain and suffering without judging or belittling ourselves.

Germer and Neff (2013) have developed a program to teach self-compassion skills to the general population. Their program demonstrated a significant increase in self-compassion, mindfulness, compassion for others, and life satisfaction along with a decrease in depression, anxiety, stress, and emotional avoidance.

Inspired by this program and based on our own experience we would like to share with you some of the ways we believe can support self-compassion while practicing medicine. Mindful awareness of shame, blame, self-flagellation, and suffering is essential in the process. As incorporated into mindfulness practice, we have to apply attitudes of acceptance and nonjudgement. We need to be familiar with our patterns of hurting and criticising ourselves.

Exercise: Self-Compassion

Notice how you treat yourself while working.
How do you perceive your mistakes and personal inadequacies?
How do you treat yourself in moments of pain and suffering? Do you ever ask yourself what you need during a busy day?
Notice the difference between how you treat a loved one and how you treat yourself when bad things happen.
When was the last time you treated yourself kindly? How did it feel?
Follow your memory and track a moment when someone you love treated you compassionately.
Let yourself be fully present with this precious situation and mindfully be aware of your body sensations, feelings, and thoughts. How does it feel?
Now, try to imagine you are this loved one who is looking at you with the same compassionate look.
What do you see? What would you like to tell yourself now?
Now, try to find your own inner compassionate voice. Find kind phrases in yourself and expand into a natural inner conversation with your compassionate voice without ignoring your inner critic voice that might arise.

For further practicing, you may try the internal metta bhavana meditation by Asaf Rolef Ben-Shahar here: www.youtube.com/watch?v=m3W_f6VXDog

5.4 Meaning

> We are here to add what we can to life, not to get what we want from life.
> —William Osler

Meaning is a human need. A deep sense of meaning strengthens us, and makes long complex hours of work tolerable. Naomi Rachel Remen (2001) emphasises the healing potential of meaning. She regards the original meaning of our work as being in service. Service for her is not a relationship between an expert and a problem; it is a human relationship, and the work of the heart and the soul. She exemplifies how meaning strengthens us not by numbing our pain or distracting us from adversity, but by reminding us of our integrity, who we are, and what we stand for. She claims it is our responsibility as healthcare providers to fight for our sense of meaning as a remedy against fatigue, numbness, and unreasonable expectations.

Although we may find ourselves busy, tired, distressed, and not fully connected, medical practice embraces abundant meaningful moments. Finding meaning will require us to see the familiar in new ways (ibid.). We do not have to rescue lives, diagnose rare diseases, or conduct heroic actions to feel a sense of meaning. Listening compassionately to a patient and being present with his suffering is very meaningful.

Rolef Ben-Shahar (2011), based on Dr. Steven Gilligan concept, emphasises the importance of a question each of us has to ask himself. He says we should ask ourselves "What does life want for me? What am I here to do?" Gilligan assumes that a good life requires active seeking of meaningfulness and further giving meaning to life.

Let us take this inquiry to medicine practice.

Why have you become a doctor?

Think of a few situations as a doctor when you felt a sense of meaning and fulfilment? How did it feel? What made those situations meaningful for you? When was the last time you felt a sense of meaning in work? Try to be mindfully attuned to moments of meaningfulness thought the day.

5.5 Somatic Resources

Somatic resources are individual physical functions, actions, and capacities, which dwell in our bodies and provide us a sense of well-being and competency (Ogden & Fisher, 2015). In this section we will discuss three fundamental, highly applicable, and efficient somatic resources derived from body psychotherapy: centring, grounding, and breathing.

1. Centring: Centring is first and foremost a stance, a way of being within oneself and in relation to the world (Rolef Ben-Shahar, 2014). It refers to regaining a sense of being connected to yourself and reconnecting with the "home" inside us (Ogden & Fisher, 2015). Centring skills—the active cultivation of minding our centre and investing in the skill to return to it, cultivating the skill of coming home—are at the heart of most body psychotherapy modalities, as well as to martial arts and other eastern physical practices (Rolef Ben-Shahar, 2014). While practicing medicine we can use centring as a way of establishing somatic awareness, strengthen our presence, and reconnect with the "home" (Ogden & Fisher, 2015, p. 309) inside us when we are thrown off balance by intricate situations.

Centring Exercise: Coming Home *(Originally presented by Rolef Ben-Shahar, 2014)*

This simple process may be used as a routine before you start working, or it may be used when you feel stressed throughout your day.

Sit comfortably and place one hand on your chest and the other on your belly, breathing effortlessly to these two regions. Stay there for a minute or two.

When breathing is as full as it can be right now, think of a time—in the distant past or recently, where you felt at home in yourself; when it was OK to be who you were just as you were; where you could stay with yourself at ease. Allow yourself to assume the posture and breathing pattern of that time, and check where you sense this inner home in your body. Let the feeling amplify.

Imagine that each breathing cycle begins in this very centre, flowing and spreading to the rest of the body, both from within to outside and from outside inwardly. Allow the breath to become a channel through which inner and outer can meet and interact.

Is there a voice that could accompany the feeling? An image? A movement? A word?

For some people, this sense could be amplified by saying sentences (either aloud or quietly) such as: "I am here, I am present, I am centred, and this is me".

2. Grounding: Grounding is a central concept in body psychotherapy, describing the body-mind interaction with its environment. It relates both to the psychological and the physiological aspects of our relationship with support and the degree of our bodily presence. It involves making an energetic and physical connection with the ground, so that energy of the body is directed downward. It fosters qualities of stability, internal security, and the ability to support ourselves and effectively use gravity (Ogden & Fisher, 2015; Rolef Ben-Shahar, 2014). This is a physical process in which we are mindfully aware of our legs and feet and their connection to the ground, directing our energy downward into the earth to sense the support of gravity (Ogden & Fisher, 2015).

Grounding Exercise

This is a useful practice (Rolef Ben-Shahar, 2014) to assist us in coming back to our bodies, strengthening our sense of bodily self and connecting to the ground. It is best done barefoot, to directly feel the contact of the body with the ground and to amplify sensory awareness. We recommend doing this exercise at the beginning of your working day.

Begin standing up straight, with the feet spread shoulder-width apart. The feet are slightly inwardly turned and knees are gently bent to avoid locking.

With the exhale, apply pressure on the feet downwards and outwards, as if trying to split the earth into two. Let go with the inhale and repeat a few times.

Add to this a gentle bending and straightening of the knees: with every inhale bend the knees, and straighten them (together with pressing down and out with the feet) with each exhale. Repeat a few times.

When there is greater energy flow to the legs, and the connection to earth is amplified, you might notice changes in body sensations, like pins and needles, streaming, vibration, or temperature changes—or even emotional shifts. Allow each of them its space with as little intervention as possible.

The last stage includes adding some sound. Repeat the process: breathing in while bending the knees, breathing out while straightening the knees and applying pressure on the earth down and out. With each exhale allow some sound to come out, ideally lower tonal registers. Repeat it for a minute or two.

Notice sensations, feelings, images, and thoughts. Notice your breathing. You may wish to walk about for a while and notice the quality of your contact with earth. Can you note differences from the beginning of the exercise? Has something in your relationship with the ground changed?

3. Breathing: Breathing is forever with us, one of the most constant forms in our life, yet at the same time, breathing is always dynamic and changing (Rolef Ben-Shahar, 2014). The way we breathe is naturally influenced by the ongoing changing circumstances. Yet, habits of breathing might affect our cognitions, emotions, and well-being. An overall pattern of relaxed, balanced breathing is thought to facilitate health and well-being (Ogden & Fisher, 2015).

Breathing exercises are among the most ancient ways of changing states of consciousness. It is one of the most efficient ways to regulate emotions, and many powerful and simple meditations use breath work. Often it is sufficient to return our attention to our breathing in order to open a fertile affective field, ripe for inner work or therapeutic work.

Breathing Exercise: Mindful Breathing

This is a simple exercise that may be used as a routine before you start working, or it may be used when you feel stressed throughout your day.

Sit comfortably and place one hand on your chest and the other on your belly.

Be mindful of your breathing. Feel your palms touch your chest and belly, feel how they move up and down with each breath.

Just be aware of your breathing moment by moment without trying to change it.

Feel your belly rise or expand gently on the inbreath, and fall or recede on outbreath.

Feel your chest rise or expand gently on the inbreath, and fall or recede on outbreath.

Focus on the various sensations associated with each breath.

How much effort is there in inspiration and expiration? How deep or shallow is your breathing? Is it fast or slow? Do you feel it mostly in your belly or in your chest?

Stay for a few more minutes with your breathing mindfully.

Breathing Exercise: Inhaling and Exhaling *(Ogden & Fisher, 2015)*

This exercise combines breath work and grounding. It may be used before you start working, or it may be used when you feel stressed throughout your day.
Sit tall in a comfortable position.
Breathe naturally and be aware of your breathing.
Breathe in fully and imagine that you pull your breath upward through the soles of your feet. Breathe out fully and imagine sending your breath down your body, through your pelvis, legs, and soles.
Repeat this breathing for a few minutes.

5.6 Self-Regulation

In the field of psychotherapy, the term *self-regulation* relates to the person's capacity to maintain systemic balance and retrieve systemic balance. We understand self-regulation as a dynamic and homeostatic phenomenon, an ongoing process of correction and adaptation (Rolef Ben-Shahar, 2014). Self-regulation is the capacity to regulating the intensity of our feelings and remain present and in contact (Carroll, 2009). It is a function of a complex system with many layers interweaving. Practicing the previously mentioned skills of grounding, centring, and breathing serve as applications of somatic self-regulation (Rolef Ben-Shahar, 2013). Being present nonjudgmentally with the whole range and intensity of our emotions, rather than avoiding them facilitates self-regulation (Carroll, 2009). For example, when I face a difficult moment with a patient and feel overwhelmed, I may become aware of my body sensations, emotions, and thoughts with acceptance and with no judgement (mindfulness), I remind myself to be self-compassionate and I use my breathing as an anchor for somatic self-regulation (reconnecting with somatic resources).

5.7 Relational Resources

As physicians, we are so used to people needing us, relying on us for knowledge, for relief, for help, and for hope. We often take this connectedness for granted, and are frequently not as good as asking for help ourselves. Yet, as poet John Donne (1839) beautifully wrote: "No man is an island, entire of itself; every man is a piece of the continent, a part of the main".

As human beings, from cradle to grave, we depend on the help and support we receive from others. When we feel accepted, valued, and supported by others we are physiologically regulated by an effect on stress hormones and various neurotransmitters (Schore, 1994, 2003).

As already discussed, practicing medicine confronts us with intricate situations, stressors, failures, and suffering. Loneliness, isolation, and lack of support are common feelings amongst doctors.

Relational resources involve our ability and willingness to communicate, reach out to others, set boundaries, give and receive emotional support. It involves setting aside the fantasy of doing it all by ourselves and learning to regulate by dialogue. There are several kinds of supportive peer groups (Epstein, 2014). Debriefing group can be described as an opportunity to meet peers and share common feelings and conflicts and get support (Gunasingam et al., 2015).

Michal Balint (1964) developed a unique discussion group that promotes exploration of the relationship between doctor and patient and allows physicians to get to know each other, discuss common issues, and support each other. More than fifty years later Balint groups exist all over the world and serve to train and develop communication skills as well as to constitute a place of sharing and support (Sklar, 2012). By taking part in a Balint group, doctors can learn to recognise personal reactions, develop an awareness of the early signals of distress, and internalise what is learnt from the interaction with other participants. They can debrief, share emotional reactions, reduce stress by sharing experiences, reinforce the value of their work, and reformulate boundaries (Benson & Magraith, 2005).

One of the basic human needs is the need for relationship. All human beings, including doctors, need to be seen, listened to, and supported. It is our responsibility to find to seek for support groups or any kind of relationship that will enable us to get the support we need and embrace us with compassionate and empathic environment.

5.8 Conclusion

The vigour of practicing medicine might become on the one hand the source of meaning, prosperity, and fulfilment, while on the other hand it might lead to exhaustion and burnout. In this chapter we have tried to highlight the valuable impact of personal disciplines of self-awareness, connecting to resources, self-care, self-compassion, and meaning all supported in a healing community of peers. The next chapter will conclude part I with clinical application of the doctor-centred medical care in practice.

References

Baker, J.A. (2003). *Caring for ourselves: A therapist's guide to personal and professional well-being.* Washington, DC: American Psychological Association.

Balint, M. (1964). *The doctor, his patient, and the illness.* London: Pitman Medical.

Benson, J., & Magraith, K. (2005). Compassion fatigue and burnout: The role of Balint groups. *Australian Family Physician, 34*(6), 497–498.

Bernard, L.K., & Curry, J.F. (2011). Self-compassion: Conceptualizations, correlates & interventions. *Review of General Psychology, 15*, 289–303.

Birnie, K., Speca, M., & Carlson, L.E. (2010). Exploring self-compassion and empathy in the context of Mindfulness-Based Stress Reduction (MBSR). *Stress and Health, 26*, 359–371.

Carroll, R. (2009). Self-regulation: An evolving concept at the heart of body psycho-therapy. In L. Hartley (Ed.), *Contemporary body psychotherapy* (pp. 89–105). Hove, East Sussex: Routledge.

Chambers, J.C., Christopher, S.E., Dunnagan, T., & Schure, M.B. (2006). Teaching self-care through mindfulness practices: The application of yoga, meditation, and qigong to counselor training. *Journal of Humanistic Psychology, 46*(4), 494–509.

Donne, J. (1839). *The Works of John Donne*. vol III. In H. Alford (ed). London: John W. Parker.

Epstein, R.M. (1999). Mindful practice. *Journal of American Medical Association, 282*(9), 833–839.

Epstein, R.M. (2014). Mindful practice. In M. Feldman & J. Christensen (Eds.), *Behavioral medicine: A guide for clinical practice* (pp. 57–63). New York, NY: McGraw Hill.

Epstein, R.M. (2017). *Attending: Medicine, mindfulness and humanity*. New York, NY: Scribner.

Gartrell, N., Milliken, N., Goodson, W.H., & Thiemann, S.B. (1992). Physician-patient sexual contact: Prevalence and problems. *Western Journal of Medicine, 157*, 139–143.

Germer, C.K. (2005). Mindfulness: What is it? What does it matter? In C. Germer, R. Siegel, & P. Fulton (Eds.), *Mindfulness and psychotherapy*. New York, NY: Guilford Press.

Germer, C.K., & Neff, K.D. (2013). Self-compassion in clinical practice. *Journal of Clinical Psychology, 69*(8), 856–867.

Gunasingam, N., Burns, K., Edwards, J., Dinh, M., & Walton, M. (2015). Reducing stress and burnout in junior doctors: The impact of debriefing sessions. *Postgraduate Medicine Journal, 91*, 182–187.

Heffernan, M., Quinn Griffin, M.T., McNulty, S.R., & Fitzpatrick, J.J. (2010). Self-compassion and emotional intelligence in nurses. *International Journal of Nursing Practice, 16*, 366–373.

Irving, J.A., Dobkin, P.L., & Park, J. (2009). Cultivating mindfulness in health care professionals: A review of empirical studies of Mindfulness-Based Stress Reduction (MBSR). *Complementary Therapies in Clinical Practice, 15*, 61–66.

Kabst-Zinn, J. (2003). Mindfulness-based interventions in context: Past, present, and future. *Clinical Psychology: Science and Practice, 10*, 144–156.

Krasner, M.S., Epstein, R.N., & Beckman, H. (2010). Association of an educational program in mindful communication with burnout, empathy, and attitudes among primary care physicians. *Journal of American Medical Association, 302*(12), 1284–1293.

Leary, M.R., Tate, E.B., Adam, C.E., Allen, A.B., & Hancock, J. (2007). Self-compassion and reactions to unpleasant self-relevant events: The implications of treating oneself kindly. *Journal of Personality and Social Psychology, 92*(5), 887–904.

McCue, J.D. (1982). The effects of stress on physicians and their medical practice. *New England Journal of Medicine, 306*, 458–463.

Meier, D.E., Back, A.L., & Morrison, S. (2001). The inner life of physicians and care of the seriously ill. *Journal of American Medical Association, 286*(23), 3007–3014.

Neff, K.D. (2003). Self-compassion: An alternative conceptualization of a healthy attitude toward oneself. *Self and Identity, 2*, 223–250.

Neff, K.D., Kirkpatrick, K.L., & Rude, S. (2007). Self-compassion and adaptive psychological functioning. *Journal of Research in Personality, 41*(1), 139–154.

Novack, D.H., Suchman, A.L., Clark, W., Epstein, R.M., Najberg, E., & Kaplan, C. (1997). Calibrating the physician: Personal awareness and effective patient care: Working group on promoting physician personal awareness: Academy on physician and patient. *Journal of American Medical Association, 278*, 502–509.

Ogden, P., & Fisher, J. (2015). *Sensorimotor psychotherapy: Intervention for trauma and attachment*. New York, NY: W.W. Norton & Co.

Pellegrino, E.D. (1993). Compassion needs reason too. *Journal of American Medical Association, 270*, 874–875.

Pick, I. (1985). Working through in the countertransference. *International Journal of Psychoanalysis, 66*, 157–166.

Remen, R.N. (2001). Recapturing the soul of medicine: Physicians need to reclaim meaning in their working lives. *Western Journal of Medicine, 174*(1), 4–5.

Rolef Ben-Shahar, A. (2011). Passion, fear and being at service. *National Register of Hypnotherapists & Psychotherapists Newsletter*, (Autumn), 10–13.

Rolef Ben-Shahar, A. (2013). The self-healing forest: Between self-regulation and dyadic regulation. *Body, Movement and Dance in Psychotherapy, 9*(1), 16–28.

Rolef Ben-Shahar, A. (2014). *Touching the relational edge: Body psychotherapy*. London: Karnac Books.

Russo, S.J., Murrough, J.W., Han, M.H., Charney, D.S., & Nestler, E.J. (2012). Neurobiology of resilience. *Nature Neuroscience, 15*(11), 1475–1484.

Schore, A. (1994). *Affect regulation and the origin of the self*. Hove, East Sussex: Lawrence Erlbaum.

Schore, A. (2003). *Affect regulation and repair of the self*. Hove, East Sussex: Lawrence Erlbaum.

Sklar, J. (2012). Regression and new beginnings: Michael, Alice and Enid Balint and the circulation of ideas. *Journal of International Psychoanalysis, 93*(4), 1017–1034.

Southwich, S.M., & Charney, D.S. (2012). *Resilience: The science of mastering life's greatest challenges*. Cambridge: Cambridge University Press.

Suchman, A.L., & Ramamurthy, G. (2014). Practitioner well-being. In M. Feldman & J. Christensen (Eds.), *Behavioral medicine: A guide for clinical practice* (pp. 51–56). New York, NY: McGraw Hill.

Weiss, L. (2004). *Therapist's guide to self-care*. New York, NY: Brunner-Routledge.

Yamey, G., & Wilkes, M. (2001). Promoting well-being among doctors. *British Medical Journal, 322*, 252–253.

Zinn, W.M. (1988). Doctors have feelings too. *Journal of American Medical Association, 259*, 3296–3298.

6 The Doctor-Centred Medical Care in Practice

In this chapter we delve into a clinical scenario illustrating the doctor-centred stance in practice. We will weave threads from each chapter using the concepts discussed and try to apply them in the medical encounter. We wish this clinical illustration will enable integration of the issues discussed and demonstrate the use of practical tools described previously.

Dizziness assails me when the nurse tells me Hanna has just called. "She wants you to come . . . again, she says she cannot breathe", the nurse informs me. It is the fifth time in two weeks that Hanna calls me. My thoughts are whirling, how can I put an end to this mess?

It was a month ago when Hanna, a seventy-year-old diabetic, hypertensive woman, came into the clinic with chest pain. It took about two minutes for her to collapse on the floor with ventricular fibrillation. It was after a successful resuscitation, and when she was finally in the ambulance escorted by sirens on her way to the hospital that I could breathe again. But it was only after a few days, when I came to see her in the hospital that I was relieved. She had no brain damage and echocardiogram showed an ejection fraction of 30% after her myocardial infarction. I was filled up with gratitude, hope, and satisfaction; it could have ended much worse. Unfortunately, Hanna did not share my feelings. While I felt gratification, she seemed frustrated and nervous every time I came to see her.

"I cannot breathe well, you have to do something", she kept saying, "The prescriptions you gave me are of no use". I have tried everything, starting with listening to her, physically examining her, consulting her cardiologist, reassuring her, and ending in discussing her fears and anxiety with her and her family. We were both trapped in this vicious cycle; every time she called me urgently telling me she cannot breathe, I came to see her, physically examined her, told her that her saturation was fine, asked her about her feelings, and she kept complaining that I was of no help for her.

And here I am now, the nurse's words surrounding me like a dust storm. I feel helpless; this mess is beyond my capability to amend.

We wish to illustrate the doctor-centred model by tracking some steps, which we have discussed in the previous chapters. These include:

1. **Don't just do something, be there**: mindfully expanding the gap between stimulus and response by realising where we are, noticing what we feel, think, and sense.
2. **Stay tuned-in**: instead of dissociating, which could provide short-term relief but in the longer term will divorce us from our resources, allow ourselves to be present with whatever we experience.
3. **Connect with resources**: Engage with skills (if these are non-existent, acquire skills) which help build up physical, mental, and emotional resources to better prepare support us with the challenge.
4. **Self-regulate**: Practice whatever skills will help us remain connected to our resourceful state. Allow ourselves to mind our needs as necessary and valid just as our patient's.
5. **Return to patient**: Once we have taken the necessary steps to care for our own emergency, attending to our needs and ensuring we have met some of them (for safety, for validation, for non-violence, for physical regulation, etc.), we can return to our patient from a different place.

These steps need not take hours. They can be practiced realistically before each patient and even during our clinical hours. But in order for these practices to be useful, they cannot only be practiced ad hoc. We need to cultivate those skills, so that when needed they would be readily available for us. Without such cultivation, they would only work sporadically, and certainly require more time than we can afford as physicians.

Please consider the following demonstration of the model. Perhaps you can appreciate that this is no magic panacea—each of these responses were worked with, cultivated, and regularly practiced.

As already discussed in the previous chapters, practicing medicine positions us in complex situations, saturated with intense emotions and challenging moments. The first step is to recognise this intricate moment and to slow down. I have to realise that I am overwhelmed, that I need to engage with my resources, to self-regulate myself, and to be mindfully aware of my feelings and needs before meeting Hanna. I choose to take a step back from my defence mechanisms (or at least to try), and instead of exorcising my feelings, dissociating, and repressing my emotions, I self-regulate myself and summon conscious coping strategies.

"I need a few moments for myself before going to Hanna", I let the nurse know. (1: Don't just do something, be there). *I feel restless and cresting like a storm wave. My heart is pounding, my breath is shallow and fast, tingling is traveling all over my body* (2: Stay tuned-in). *I let my attention go to my feet and pelvis, and I am mindful to the support of gravity and my connection to*

earth (grounding). *I observe my breath mindfully while putting one hand on my chest and the other on my belly* (3: Connect with resources: centring and breathing). *The warmth of my hand wraps my chest softly, I calm down* (4: Self regulate). *Startled by feeling angry and bereft of humanness towards Hanna, a mix of guilt, sadness, and disappointment is emerging. My heart is open again. I can now turn my attention back to Hanna and be there fully* (5: Return to patient—please note that I continue to monitor myself even during the interaction with Hanna).

Hanna is sitting in her couch when I come in. She strides haughtily towards her bedroom, gazing at me with derision. Dead silence takes after a waterfall of complaining words pour out from her. Intimidated by her presence, my heart is beating light and rapid, my muscles are contracted, I feel like a scolded child (mindful self-awareness, 1 & 2). *I take a few breaths, strengthen my back, and remind myself of the good moments Hanna and I used to have once* (connecting to somatic, emotional, and cognitive resources, 3 & 4).

I am looking into her brown eyes; restrained anger coiled through her obstinate gaze strikes me.

"You are angry at me . . ." I am suddenly saying. Her eyes are widened when she slumps on her seat.

"I am very angry at you", she says loudly after a few seconds of hesitation. "It is your entire fault, you know", she keeps talking furiously. "All this suffering . . . for what? I should have died that day, if it weren't for your silly efforts. How dare you come and tell me I am OK? I will never forgive you . . . as long as I live, I will make you miserable".

Her words punch me in the chest (1). *Stunned and humiliated I close my eyes for a moment. Clenching my fists, anger is spreading throughout my body interwoven with shame and self-flagellation* (mindful self-awareness, 2). *I use my breath as an anchor so I can stay fully present, trying to be kind to myself and accept my feelings with no judgement as far as possible* (connecting to somatic resources and self-compassion, 3 & 4). *Beyond her enraged gaze I can see her agony. Rage and wrath blend with sorrow and grief. Pain lodges in my chest; my heart is open again.*

Taking a few minutes break before going to Hanna was crucial. Recognising my distress and being aware of my basic needs enabled me to self-regulate and cultivate my well-being. These are prerequisites for mindful practice and empathic communication. Observing my body sensations and intense emotions, I notice my overwhelming feelings. Instead of being identified with the emotional flooding, reacting emotionally or dissociating, I choose to connect with somatic resources such as grounding, centring, and breathing, and to self-regulate myself. Calmed down, I have the capacity to mindfully be aware of a full range of emotions that shed light on my understanding of this intricate situation. I endeavour to do it curiously, non-judgmentally with acceptance and self-compassion. Attuned to myself, aware of my feelings, resourced and self-regulated, my attention to Hanna's feelings broadens and gets clearer. Hanna reminds me of how habitual and prevailing my tendency to push away Hanna's suffering and embellish my medical success is. After a long time of my denial of her anger and suffering, I am capable of recognising it and talking about it while being fully present. Attending to Hanna's suffering is not an easy choice. I have to face my own fears, vulnerability, and helplessness. I have to take responsibility for my incapability to be present with the various aspects of her suffering. I have to remind myself that engaging with difficult situations instead of withdrawing fosters well-being. I engage with the original meaning of being a doctor. Being in service not only as an expert and a life saviour, but also being in a human relationship, listening and supporting the heart and the soul.

"It must be so hard . . ." I whisper, looking at her. Her eyes glitter like broken glass, when she hears me saying, "I am so sorry . . . I didn't know". I can feel seeds of tears behind my eyes. Her body softens. She dissolves into tears when she painfully says, "I am so lonely". I put my hand on her shoulder and we endure her sorrow and pain together.

Part II

The Doctor-Patient Relationship, Exercising Therapeutic Skills Without Being a Psychotherapist

7 The Complexity of the Doctor-Patient Relationship

> But a moment comes, at it is near, when the shuddering man looks up and sees both pictures in a flash together. And a deeper shudder seizes him.
>
> —Martin Buber (1958), p. 72

The doctor-patient relationship is the foundation of medical care. The medical encounter brings together two experts: the doctor whose expertise is making diagnosis and conducting treatment, and the patient whose expertness is his own history, experience, and insights regarding his medical state, functionality, and quality of life (Roter & Hall, 2006). However, the medical encounter also constitutes a meeting between two human beings with their own expectations, needs, stereotypes, and biographies. When these two relationships manage to meet creatively and benevolently, healing can occur, but moreover, our humanity received affirmation and we reach a special place, perhaps that very deeper shudder of which Buber speaks of.

Tauber (1999) describes the doctor-patient relationship as based on a shared understanding of illness, while the doctor does not only serve as an objective observer, but also participates in a partnership with his patient. He also notes the magnitude of responsibility, commitment, empathy, and the doctor's personality as the ground of the doctor-patient relationship.

While there is no doubt in regard of its paramount influence on the medical encounter, the doctor-patient relationship carries a myriad of intricacies and complexities. Medical care has been changing tremendously throughout the past decades. Polarities between scientific medicine and humanity together with the disparity between autonomy and authority in the doctor-patient relationship are significant factors in the shift in this challenging relationship over the last years (Mitchell, 2005)

In this chapter we will discuss and elaborate those issues and their influence on our clinical work by interweaving theory and clinical experience.

7.1 Objectivity and Subjectivity in Medicine

Western medicine has evolved in a tradition of empiricism and realism where scientific and experimental methodology is highly appreciated (Little, 1995).

Initiated in the 17th century with contributions from Newton and Descartes, traditional science was rooted with an objectivist philosophy, affecting the essence of medical practice (Cassell, 1997). The post–World War II era has been addressed to as a preponderant time for modern medicine (Shorter, 1985). The drug revolution, originated in the discovery of sulfa drugs and penicillin, led medicine towards a scientific-oriented expertise and gave birth to the "biomedical" model of disease (Roter & Hall, 2006). While the scientific revolution has yielded great achievements in medical care, it has complexly influenced the doctor-patient relationship. The empirical objective approach has captured the traditional ethos of medicine, reinforcing the patient's objectification (Tauber, 1999). The patient afflicted with an illness turned into a case of a syndrome or condition (Toulmin, 1993), and doctors came to recognise themselves as possessing a new power, enabling them to discern the mysterious of nature and diseases (Tauber, 1999). Notwithstanding the scientific triumph and achievements, both patients and doctors have been increasingly confronted with medicine's failure to address many ailments, and with necessary scrutiny with regard to claims and promises of scientific medicine. Without diminishing the huge progress attributed to scientific approach, it has also made patients become diseased bodies exemplifying some pathological entity (Tauber, 1999; Toulmin, 1993). In essence, like many similar scientific and human revolutions, we have been called to humbly acknowledge our innate limitations.

A few years ago I happened to attend an ultrasound exam of a pregnant woman conducted by a colleague of mine. When this young, ambitious, and skilled doctor diagnosed a rare malformation in the fetus, he was so satisfied and enthusiastic that he had totally forgotten the devastating meaning for his patient.

We all want to be excellent doctors; inculcated with an objectivist stance, we seek for more knowledge of diseases, diagnoses, guidelines, skills, and clinical evidence. Whereas the power of science has bred enormous success, it has also given rise to alienation from humanity. Tauber (1999) claims that we can no longer overlook the fact that the application of scientific medicine is only one aspect of medical care, and calls for empathy and emotional support that recognises psychological needs and cultural aspects as factors that have to be understood to effectively treat patients. He further argues that as doctors we cannot perceive ill patients as isolated objects, but must consider them in a broader and complex array of suffering.

We have been witnessing in the past years a shift away from objectivist and realistic stances toward a more subjectivist paradigm, a context-sensitive model where relationality and observer's subjectivity have become acceptable (Wilson, 2000). In medical literature there has been more interest in the last decades in researching humanity in medicine and the doctor-patient relationship, with considerable support affirming their significant impact on the outcome of the medical encounter (Arafat et al., 2017; Bass et al., 1986; Kaplan et al., 1989; Spiro, 1992; Stewart, 1995). The biopsychosocial approach which views illness and health as a result of an interaction between biological, psychological, and social factors, and underscores humanity and empathy, has emerged from dissatisfaction with the biomedical model. This more holistic model of illness has been incorporated by medical specialists, researched, and validated (Epstein, 2017; Wade & Halligan, 2017).

This growing evidence defies and challenges the realistic epistemological basis of the biomedical model, that the doctor can be an observer without influencing the one who is observed (Wilson, 2000). That is to say, our human presence has impact on our patients. In discussing therapeutic influence versus the importance of the patient's autonomy, psychoanalyst Stephen Mitchell (2004) argued that the analyst's own biography and emotional states, as these manifested in the therapeutic relationship were not only inevitable but also essential for the therapeutic process. He succinctly wrote: "There is no way to filter out the analyst's impact on the process" (p. 540).

Since the medical encounter is based on a relationship between two people with an inner life, we would further say, that doctors and patients influence each other. Recognising this mutual influence and its impact would affect the care we provide.

Mitchell (1997) distinguishes between science and scientism. The former refers to the accumulation of knowledge in certain methods, while the latter refers to the belief that such knowledge has the ultimate answers regarding the human experience. He observes that whereas science continues to advance, scientism has faded. He warns against the phenomena of replacing objectivism by a total subjectivism where science loses its impact. He believes that the problem has not been science itself, but scientism that has inflated our expectations of science and made us mistakenly believe that it will provide us with answers to most of our questions. Scientism, which is in effect a form of religion, in the placing of all knowledge and truth within a reductive system, has given us authority as the owners of powerful knowledge leading to paternalistic models of relationships with our patients. The fading scientism and the call for subjectivism have abated our authority and cracked the paternalistic model.

This is a challenging time for us as doctors. We are in the middle of a revolution in providing medical care. We are expected to be scientific and objective, as well as remain human and caring (Bensing et al., 2006; Tauber, 1999). We have to serve our patients while interweaving dexterity and finesse, science and the art of healing, while our privileged status as owners of the power of knowledge has been cracked, and we can no longer enjoy the autonomy we used to own. Dr. Google has replaced the authority which was once projected upon us, and we wish to suggest that while introducing complex and sometimes uncomfortable dynamics into the doctor-patient relationship, it also provides us with opportunity to practice humanely, and to find expertise in humble practice rather than pretentiously holding a position of omniscience. These issues raise questions regarding the nature of our knowledge and authority, the relationship between contemporary medicine and the classical tradition, and what we have to offer our patients nowadays.

7.2 Autonomy and Authority, the Power of the White Coat

I admired him. We all did. Looking up to him, as a little girl, he was like a God to me. Standing up with his white coat and a serious expression on his face; operating peculiar instruments; and always knowing the answers.

He was my father's doctor.

His words were sanctified and I believed everything he said. Operation, chemotherapy, and radiation . . . whatever he said . . . We had no doubt, no internet, and no other sources of information. It was just him. We entrusted him with my father's life. And he did it . . . Time and again he did his miracles and saved his life.

Years have passed; I have become a doctor myself. The divine appearance has been cracked; uncertainty and the limits of medical science have been striking me. There are plenty of data resources, patients no longer hesitate to ask questions, they demand to know more, they wish to choose and decide. At the same time, as my father's daughter, I ask his doctors questions, I want to hear about possible options and their consequences, and to let him decide. The admiring naïve little girl has turned into a realistic daughter (and doctor) who believes in taking charge of one's life and make own choices.

And then it happens . . . My father is in the operating room with perforation of his colon, when the doctor comes out. "It's all a mess in there, I am sorry. His pancreatic tumour has spread out", he says. "There are two options. We can either repair the colon perforation, or we can let him die . . . Your decision to make ". My heart is racing, I can hardly breathe, and my legs are becoming weak. He is staring at me, waiting for my decision. I look at him, my father's doctor. And for a few seconds I am desperately looking for the God-doctor, the one that can perform miracles, the one that knows what's best, the one that I can fully trust to decide for me. I feel fuzzy, as if my brain has stopped.

How can I decide?

I take a few breaths, I close my eyes for a second, "let him die", I say.

What sort of expertise do we have as doctors? What is the kind of knowledge and authority we claim for us? What is our role as physicians? To what extent should we enable our patients' autonomy to decide medical decisions?

When a patient comes to see a doctor, he grants authority and expertise to him. Our long training, cumulative knowledge, and clinical experience delegate that authority and expertise.

Until recently the doctor's knowledge and authority went hand in hand. The scientific knowledge gave us the authority to express our definite understandings about our patients' medical conditions and forward our recommendations. Patients had to accept medical practice on faith, protected by doctors' high code of moral conduct.

Parallel to the scientific revolution, we have been facing another transformation by the rise of Western liberalism, relocating the authority of decision making to the individual. This principle of patient autonomy and self-determination is a doctrine that recognises the patient's right (and duty) to take an active role in treatment decision making (Chin, 2002; Schneider, 1998). The decreasing difference in knowledge between doctors and patients (Lo & Parham, 2010; McMullan, 2006) associated with fading scientism and the rising the principle of autonomy, have made patients more active in medical decision making, and more confident in their ability to manage their diseases (Murray et al., 2003). Therefore, after centuries of being allowed to overrule patients' preferences with the aim of protecting patients and preventing harm, doctors no longer receive unquestioned acceptance as the dominant mode for decision-making in medical care (Chin, 2002). The traditional prototype of paternalism, in which the physician functions as a professionally dominant and autonomous guardian and the patient's role is passive and dependent, has been mostly replaced by a model of mutuality. In this model, which is based on the principle of patient autonomy, both doctors and patients bring strengths and resources to the relationship, and decisions are the result of negotiation between both (Fritzsche et al., 2014; Roter & Hall, 2006). The autonomy paradigm has brought about the magnitude of empowerment of patients' rights to be informed, make choices, be responsible for accepting medical risks, and take charge for their own health (Funnel, 2000; Roter & Hall, 2006). It had also freed the physicians (or forced them) to be more human.

Alongside its outstanding advantages, the growing autonomy of the patient in medical care has rendered a myriad of concerns and complexities. The main concerns attributed to this shift from medical paternalism to patient autonomy relate to the power dynamics, mutuality, and asymmetry between patients and doctors. Power relations in the medical encounter are articulated through three main elements: (1) who sets the agenda and goals; (2) the role of the patient's values; (3) the doctor's relational approach. Each medical attitude generates its own power dynamics and impacts the quality of the working alliance. Tauber (1999) remarks that arguing for the mutual model does not mean that this relationship is symmetrical. He further elaborates that there is no parity between roles of the doctor and his patient. He asserts that since patients lack the training and knowledge to make complex medical decisions, they cannot have full autonomy. He foregrounds how judgement is crucial in making decisions and alludes us that when we are sick, we might lose our capacity for objectivity. Chin (2002) contributes to the subject by pointing out the threats of eclipsing the principle of medical beneficence. He wonders whether medicine can "continue to serve the patient if cleansed totally of parental motivation" (p. 152). He designates that there are patients that are not prepared for absolute autonomy and may be best served by a model called "guided paternalism" (Elwyn et al., 1999) which strives to augment and optimise the patient's autonomy.

How can we hold the tension between mutuality and asymmetry? How can we interweave our expertise with the recognition of patient autonomy for the sake of beneficence of our patients?

To explore the balance between these polarities (expertise vs. autonomy, mutuality vs. asymmetry) more fully, we shall later introduce you to this dilemma as it was discussed in the field of psychotherapy, primarily relational psychoanalysis.

7.3 A Mindful Doctor-Patient Relationship

We can begin by asserting an obvious, but often forgotten assumption: the question of doctor-patient relationship, and the extent to which we pay interest to it, should be in direct correlation with patient's well-being. That is, the quality of the relationship is recognised as an important factor for the benefit of the patient, and we attempt to monitor it by raising some of these questions: How do we increase patient cooperation? How do we ensure implementation of doctor's orders? How do we encourage the patient's responsibility for their health and well-being? How can the doctor-patient relationship become a benevolent (and when is it malevolent) agent in recovery and healing? These questions and others guide are context-sensitive, they depend on the culture, class, age, gender, power, and privilege, as well as many other factors. If we wish to maximise the efficacy and quality of the healthcare we provide, we need to take these factors into account.

The pendulum between medical authority and patient autonomy is complex and influenced by both patient's and doctor's parameters. Patient's social world, physical condition, and character, together with doctor's point of view, values, and personality are relevant for the kind of relationship that is formed. There has been a profound discussion in the medical literature regarding these intricacies and complexities. Most would point out there is no need to make an absolute discernment between paternalism and autonomy, and prefer one over another (Chin, 2002; Devettere, 2000; Roter & Hall, 2006; Tauber, 1999). Applying an approach that integrates the motivation of doing good for the patient, together with the recognition of patient's responsibility and freedom to make decisions enhanced by physician's advice, is challenging. This attitude calls for our integrity, morality, and flexibility (Roter & Hall, 2006; Tauber, 1999).

However, this is a tricky issue that asks for self-awareness of the effects and impact which our stance, values, and personality have on patients' autonomy. And because medicine, to a great extent, relied on the expert-god model for decades, which 'freed' the physicians of the need to face their limited humanity, and similarly 'liberated' the patients from the need to take responsibility of their own health, by providing them with an omniscience godlike figure.

One aspect that deserves a thoughtful discourse is the fact that each one of us has his own idiosyncratic style of relating to patients. Some of us naturally incline to be more authoritarian and paternalistic, while others feel more comfortable with exercising a more permissive communication, giving patients full autonomy in the process of decision making. As we have already mentioned, as doctors we need to be flexible with our attitude and wander between both edges according to our patients' needs and conditions. Being mindful and self-aware to the way we tend to relate is of paramount importance: it allows us to respect our needs, to be better aware of our impact, and at the same time such self-awareness provides us with a plethora of opportunities to expand and grow our skills. While teaching young doctors communication skills, we encourage mindfully exploring each one's tendency and experiencing different attitudes. Based on our experience flexibility is cultivated by self-awareness and mindful practice.

Another noteworthy aspect is recognising the impact we have on patients resulted by our human presence and the way we communicate. The following example would illustrate our point. A young, pregnant woman infected with Cytomegalovirus comes to her gynaecologist for consultation. The doctor presents her with the relevant information, explains her risks and options based on his medical knowledge, and gives her the possibility to make her choice. He may conduct the medical encounter with a concerned utterance, emphasising the risks and the fact that she is healthy and young to have other babies, or he can be calm, underscoring the little chance of the fetus to be infected, and the efficacy of prenatal diagnosis. While in both cases he shares his knowledge with the patient and promotes her autonomy, his own values and personality significantly influence the patient's decision. Ignoring our unconscious messages in the medical encounter and underestimating our profound influence on the process of decision making, have the potential of making us unintentionally self-deceivers. To allow our patient genuine informed decisions, we need to be mindful of what beliefs, values, and emotional attitudes we convey in our communication.

Psychoanalyst Steven Mitchell (1997) argues that the patient's autonomy is more honestly and meaningfully preserved through acknowledgement of our influence rather than through pleading to illusory objectivity. In his attempt to formulate psychoanalysis as a science, Freud aspired to create a value-free psychotherapy, as clean as possible from the therapist's influence. From its inception, psychoanalysis has always placed the greatest importance on the patient's autonomy and self-direction. Nevertheless, today it is widely accepted that influence, not least therapeutic influence, is unavoidable. Psychotherapist Bradford Keeney (1983) reiterated a similar position: "Therapists affect the systems they are treating whether they intend to or not. On the other side of the relationship, the systems treated always affect the therapist" (p. 129). After many decades of laborious attempts to eradicate, or at least minimise, the therapist's influence on the patient (and vice versa), modern psychoanalysis now recognises that such attempts are not only illusory and impossible, but they moreover hinder the healing and curative quality of a relationship (Mitchell, 1997). We are not expected to be without impact or influence. Instead, we are called to take responsibility and become familiar with our impact and influence, to cultivate sensitivity to these issues.

The role of physicians has changed today. We have abdicated the omnipotent godlike position of holding knowledge, decision, and execution in favour of service providers and advocates. The basic percept of the physician is to care for the patient by sharing knowledge, decision making, and choices with respect for the individual's autonomy. We believe that self-awareness and recognition of our influence on patients are essential for cultivating integrity, morality, and flexibility in medical care. When doctor and patient come together, each affects the experience of the other. Each relationship is unique and informed by the conscious and unconscious reactions, values, and personalities of each.

References

Arafat, Y., Kabir, R., & Andalib, A. (2017). A narrative review on progression of doctor-patient relationship model in light of time and culture. *International Journal of Perceptions in Public Health, 1*(2), 102–107.

Bass, M.J., Buck, C., & Turner, L. (1986). The physicians' actions and the outcome of illness in family practice. *Journal of Family Practice, 23*, 43–47.

Bensing, J., Tromp, F., Van Dulmen, S., Van den Brink-Muinen, A., Verheul, W., & Schellevis, F. (2006). Shifts in doctor-patient communication between 1986 and 2002: A study of videotaped general practice consultations with hypertension patients. *Family Practice, 7*, 62–68.

Buber, M. (1958). *I and Thou* (R.G. Smith, Trans.). New York, NY: Scribner.

Cassell, E. (1997). *Doctoring: The nature of primary care medicine*. New York, NY: Oxford University Press.

Chin, J.J. (2002). Doctor-patient relationship: From medical paternalism to enhanced autonomy. *Singapore Medical Journal, 43*(3), 152–155.

Devettere, R.J. (2000). *Practical decision making in health care ethics: Cases and concepts* (2nd ed.). Washington, DC: Georgetown University Press.

Elwyn, G., Edwards, A., Gwyn, R., & Grol, R. (1999). Towards a feasible model for shared decision making: Focus group study with general practice registrars. *British Medical Journal, 391*, 753–756.

Epstein, E. (2017). *Attending: Medicine, mindfulness and humanity*. New York, NY: Scribner.

Funnell, M.M. (2000). Helping patients take charge of their chronic illnesses. *Family Practice Management, 7*(3), 47–51.

Fritzsche, K., Schweickhardt, A., Frahm, G., Diaz Monsalve, S., Afshar Zanjani, H., & Goli, F. (2014). Doctor-patient communication. In K. Fritzsche, S.H. McDaniel, & M. Wirsching (Eds.), *Psychosomatic medicine: An international primer for the primary care setting*. New York; Heidelberg; Dordrecht; London: Springer.

Kaplan, S.H., Greenfield, S., & Ware, J.E. (1989). Assessing the effects of physician-patient interactions on the outcomes of chronic disease. *Medical Care, 275*, 5110–5127.

Keeney, B. (1983). *Aesthetics of change*. New York, NY: Guilford Press.

Little, J.M. (1995). *Humane medicine*. Cambridge: Cambridge University Press.

Lo, B., & Parham, L. (2010). The impact of Web 2.0 on the doctor-patient relationship. *Journal of Law and Medical Ethics, 38*(1), 17–26.

McMullan, M. (2006). Patients using the internet to obtain health information: How this affects the patient-health professional relationship. *Patient Education Counseling, 63*, 24–28.

Mitchell, S.A. (1997). *Influence and autonomy in psychoanalysis*. Hillsdale, NJ: Analytic Press.

Mitchell, S.A. (2004). My psychoanalytic journey. *Psychoanalytic Inquiry, 24*(4), 531–541.

Murray, E., Lo, B., Pollack, L., Donelan, K., Catania, J., & White, M. (2003). The impact of health information on the inter-net on the physician-patient relationship: Patient perceptions. *Archives of Internal Medicine, 163*, 1727–173.

Roter, D.L., & Hall, J.A. (2006). *Doctors talking with patients/ patients talking with doctors: Improving communication in medical visits.* Westport, CT: Praeger Publishers.

Schneider, C.E. (1998). *The practice of autonomy: Patients, doctors, and medical decisions.* New York, NY: Oxford University Press.

Shorter, E. (1985). *Bedside manners.* New York, NY: Simon and Schuster.

Spiro, H. (1992). What is empathy and can it be taught? *Annals of Internal Medicine, 116*, 843–846.

Stewart, M.A. (1995). Effective physician-patient communication and health outcomes: A review. *Canadian Medical Association Journal, 152*, 1423–1433.

Tauber, A.I. (1999). *Confessions of a medicine man: An essay in popular philosophy.* Cambridge, MA: Massachusetts Institute of Technology Press.

Toulmin, S. (1993). Knowledge and art in the practice of medicine. In C. Delkeskamp-Hayes & M. Cutler (Eds.), *Science, technology and the art of medicine.* New York, NY: Kluwer Academic.

Wade, D.T., & Halligan, P.W. (2017). The biopsychosocial model of illness: A model whose time has come. *Clinical Rehabilitation, 31*(8), 995–1004.

Wilson, H.J. (2000). The myth of objectivity: Is medicine moving towards a social constructivist medical paradigm? *Family Practice, 17*, 203–209.

8   The Patient

Transference and Regressive Self-States[1]

The foundation of healthcare is the therapeutic alliance, whereby patient and doctor come together with their expectations and try to establish rapport which supports the treatment. Some of the expectations are determined by realistic perceptions, and some are associated and affected by our past, anxiety, and neediness.

Let us look at the following three examples:

Lisa is a sixty-year-old diabetic woman. She has much respect and appreciation for her doctor. She trusts him and follows his recommendations without any doubt. She is one of the most compliant patients, always nice and thankful. From time to time she brings her family physician a small present.

Jenny is a thirty-five-year-old mother. She comes to the paediatrician with her six-year-old daughter, who has fever and has been coughing for a couple of days. She demands prescription for antibiotics even though the doctor has diagnosed a viral upper respiratory tract infection. She does not trust doctors; she never will. She tends to be impatient and demanding, and she is hard to satisfy. Life has taught her to rely only on herself. After doctors had missed her mother's tumour, she decided to take responsibility and be in charge of health issues.

John is a fifty-five-year-old executive director, recovering from a recent, extensive myocardial infarction. In contrast to his high functionality at work, he comes to his family physician anxious and helpless. He suffers from mild depression associated with anxiety. He finds it difficult to make decisions regarding his health, and he needs his doctor to tell him what to do.

We are all familiar with these patients. Each presents different expectations, attitudes, and behaviour. When patients come to their doctors they tend to see what they expect to see, and behave accordingly. By doing that they give subtle non-explicit messages about the part they are playing, and invite doctors to adopt the role or behaviour that is expected (Hughes & Kerr, 2000; Ryle, 1998).

In this chapter we will present psychological phenomena of transference, regression, and projective identification. We will discuss those issues and their relevance and implications in medical care. We will focus on the patient's experience in the dynamics of the doctor-patient relationship. We believe that awareness and understanding of these phenomena will shed light on the complexity of the medical encounter and cultivate better communication and rapport.

8.1 Transference

Anywhere we go, and no matter how intelligent we are, we take all our previous relationships with us. Within us we carry our mothers and fathers, our siblings and our doctors and teachers. Past experiences, particularly from our formative years, are the lenses through which we now view relationships. These lenses are not merely passive filters; instead these are active agents in contributing to the manner in which we create new relationships and position ourselves within them—both now and in the future. If our primary school headmaster was frightening and authoritarian, we are more likely to respond to our children's headmaster with apprehension and dis-ease. We learn genderial roles and expectations early on and act upon them later on in life. A great deal of our relationships and communication is tainted by our past relating.

Transference is an unavoidable psychological phenomenon in which we unconsciously transfer feelings and attitudes from a person in our past on to a person in the present situation (Hughes & Kerr, 2000). In other words, our early experiences of relating and interacting seriously influence the way in which we relate to others as adults. These previous relationships provide us with lenses through which we look at later relationships in our lives. At the heart of transference dynamics lays a simple assumption: our past influences our present. We relate to others not merely by noticing who they are, but also by applying our previous experience on the current situation. Transference becomes complex when our past experiences lead us to behave in ways that are either unhelpful for us, or harmful to others. Transference phenomena are not unique to psychotherapy or medicine: they are everywhere, a mark of the incredible human capacity to learn from experience, to form habitual patterns that free our minds to deal with other things.

Psychoanalyst Harry Stack Sullivan (1954) illustrated it thus: "Even though only two people are actually in the room, the number of more or less imaginary people that get themselves involved in this two-group is sometimes really hair-raising" (pp. 8–9). We believe that transference dynamics cannot but be part of relationships; that transferential dynamics are inevitable since we relate to the world through our previous experience of the selves we have partaken in—we were created in relationships and bring those remembered selves into any new connection.

While each relationship includes transferential components, the more emotionally or physically challenging the situation, the more reactive we become and, hence, the more powerful transference-dynamics become. Since visits to the doctor are imbued with pain, hope, fear, and helplessness, the doctor-patient relationship is particularly prone for certain transference patterns (Hughes & Kerr, 2000)—and for highly amplified transference responses. Our patients mostly don't see the person behind the white coat; they see someone who can help them, someone who helps them, or someone who 'refuses' to help. They see the doctors they had as children and other authoritative figures.

Can we, as physicians, genuinely argue that we see them more clearly than they see us?

When doctor and patient meet, they both bring their biographies to the relationship. For example, one might relate his doctor with the same terror and fear he used to feel towards his dominant and threatening father. That is to say, that transference is promoted by unconscious expectations related to the lenses through which we perceive our doctor; hence distortions might take place in the patient's apprehension of an interaction.

The situation of neediness and dependence on the doctor together with the therapeutic setting, where patients are seen frequently, makes this complex relationship of doctor and patient saturated with intense feelings, fears, vulnerability, expectations, and hopes. It is of paramount importance for us to recognise that as doctors we might become significant attachment figures for patients. As such, patients transfer a myriad of thoughts, feelings, hopes, and desires that are not necessarily connected to us (Fritzsche et al., 2014). These are rooted in patients' biographies, character traits, and cultural and gender factors, and aggravated by the characteristics of the medical encounter. To reiterate—to recognise and realise that the person our patients fear, desire, reach out to, admire—is seldom completely us. One of the most important aspects of psychotherapeutic training, and a principle which we believe is crucial for physicians to practice too, is not to take things too personally—neither good ones, nor bad ones. How to balance this not taking things too personally together with professional rigour and assuming proper responsibility is indeed an art which requires experience, maturity, and understanding.

Let us look at the asymmetrical nature of the doctor-patient relationship and its influence on transference dynamics. As elaborated in the previous chapter, doctors hold the power of knowledge which provides them with authority to some degree and influence on the patient. Moreover, the patient is waiting for the doctor, meaning that the doctor's time is more precious; the patient is weak, ill, needy, and dependent, while the doctor represents healthiness and strength; the patient meets his doctor, with none of his accomplishments and skills that make him feel self-worth, while his doctor's white coat awards him with his respectful professionalism. Each patient will react differently within such asymmetric dynamics.

In the examples given at the beginning of the chapter we can observe three patterns of common transference dynamics.

Lisa tends to idealise her doctor and see him as a wise and caring parent. While this kind of relationship often promotes compliance and trust, it may also enhance paternalistic dynamics dominating the doctor and abating the patient's autonomy.

Jenny transfers feelings of anger, mistrust, and dissatisfaction on her doctor as a result of her previous experience with medical system. Because she is very worried and anxious, perceiving her doctor as unreliable and defiant, she comes to the medical encounter in order to fight for her daughter's life. This kind of attitude encourages confrontations and clashes between doctors and patients.

John projects a needed aspect of a previously experienced or wished relationship on to his doctor. His anxiety and neediness provoked by his recent myocardial infarction make him adopt a helpless child-like role and perceive his doctor as an omnipotent parent that is expected to provide him with solutions. This kind of relationship might deepen his dependence and hinder the process of taking charge of his illness.

As we can see, numerous of patients' feelings, emotions, attitudes, and behaviours towards their doctors are unconsciously projected on to them affecting the therapeutic relationship. Instead of doctors' tendency to take these attitudes personally, it can be considered as patients' way to communicate their needs that are not verbally expressed. Nonetheless, we have to beware of making transference our defence against patients' vindicated feelings towards us. Our unintentional mistakes, failures, and insensitivity might justify our patients' anger. While some of transference feelings do not impede treatment, some might dominate the relationship and impair appropriate management (Hughes & Kerr, 2000). In these cases awareness and recognition of transferential feelings are of paramount importance for understanding better patient's agenda, expectations, and needs; communicating; and planning clinical management.

8.2 Projective Identification

Rachel suffered from severe migraines as a child. Her parents and doctors were certain this was merely a way to avoid going to school. Nobody believed her. Her experience showed that only by manipulation and exaggeration she could get people to truly hear what she experienced. As she arrives to the clinic, she starts telling a very long story. It feels made up, and the physician starts moving uncomfortably in her chair. She asks Rachel some questions, and Rachel, who notices her doctor's looks, begin to behave even more extremely, which in turn makes her physician more suspicious.

A self-fulfilling prophecy, projective identification is a theatre of past experiences projected upon the present and enacted to justify its validity.

Projective identification is an unconscious process whereby one person projects his inner feelings on another person. In response to the projection, the other person behaves in accordance with the projected feeling. Recognising the phenomenon could help us disentangle from its grip. For instance, the physician noticing her increasing distrust may approach Rachel and say, "it's not easy to believe that you can communicate exactly what you are going through," which could dissipate the transference-tie. To be able to respond like that depends on the physician's familiarity with her own feelings and reactions, and not taking her patient's behaviours too personally. Another common scenario is a feeling of fatigue, low energy, and hopelessness when meeting a depressive patient. For example, Mathew comes to a doctor complaining of low back pain. In his past, every time he was in pain—nobody could really help. Everybody withdrew from him as a child and he believes that his difficulty is too much for anybody. In the clinical interview, the doctor suddenly feels hopeless and weary and he lacks his usual energy. Mathew notices his physician stifling a yawn, and feels even more depressed and helpless, which in turn activates the doctor's difficulty even more. Recognising the shift in his inner experience when meeting his patient, the doctor can use it as an important piece of information regarding his patient. Based on this information he might take an extensive psychosocial anamnesis and ask him depressive screening questions.

It is important to emphasise that the aim of projective identification is to enhance affective communication and to evoke empathy and understanding as well as to assure a container outside of oneself who would hold and manage the unwanted feelings. That is, our patients do not tell us what they are going through, they actually show us—through their behaviour and its immediate impact on us. In fact, this unconscious process is often considered the psychobiological foundation of empathy (Rothschild & Rand, 2006). Being aware of this unconscious psychological phenomenon in the medical encounter might help us better understand our patient's feelings, rather than reacting and behaving out of identification with them. It would enrich our comprehension of complex situations and help us better communicating with our patients.

8.3 Regressive Self-States

Rubens is a functional and intelligent, self-employed man. He is married and father to three teenage children. He is also diabetic; he seems to be wise and eloquent; he is unresponsive to treatment. He consumes sugary food, does not do any physical activity, and avoids taking responsibility for his condition. In his doctor appointments, he either excessively lies or complains like a child, begging me to help him with utter helplessness. He doesn't feel like a man, but instead like a small boy who is being naughty and then feeling guilty for his behaviour.

Have you ever treated an adult patient who was acting like a child? Have you wondered what could have caused it?

Regression is considered a defence mechanism in which one returns to a childlike self-state. It is a form of retreat whereby one goes back to a time when one felt safer, or where an all-powerful parent would take the child away. This unconscious psychological phenomenon involves taking the position of a child in an intricate situation, rather than acting in an adult way, and it happens within a relational context; that is, regression is a form of transference. Where there is a child, there is also a parent. Regression is often evoked in response to stressful situations. Since the medical encounter encompasses stressful situations together with asymmetric relationship and certain transference dynamics, it is a fertile soil for regressive self-states formation. The patient 'becomes' young and relates to the doctor as the parent or the responsible adult. One patient might express his regression with a "temper tantrum" in response to waiting for long time for his doctor when he feels bad. Another one would act like a helpless child when he is ill expecting the doctor to "save" him.

Regressive behaviour might be simple and harmless, but it can also be more dysfunctional and impairing medical management by affecting communication, expectations, compliance, and the process of sharing medical decisions and taking charge of one's own illness. As discussed earlier in the chapter, John's anxiety and neediness provoked by his recent myocardial infarction, made him revert to a regressive self-state as a helpless child that perceives his doctor as an omnipotent parent that is expected to "save" him and provide him with solutions. When John expresses his regressive behaviour, he communicates his anxiety, helplessness, and neediness.

As doctors we may respond to child states in several ways consciously or unconsciously. We might take a parent position of authority in which nurturing and controlling are dominant, or we might call forth an adult state of our patient. We might revel in the patient's admiration and fail to recognise the dangerous power-dynamics therein. As we have already mentioned, regressive states might be innocuous as well as detrimental. We have to beware of adopting automatically an omnipotent therapeutic position, which could burden the patient and the medical care with difficulties (Rolef Ben-Shahar, 2014; Totton, 2003). There are times, especially in an acute crisis, where taking the role of an omnipotent parent would serve beneficently our patient, while in other times, it would deepen the patient's regressive behaviour fostering dependence, dysfunction, unrealistic expectations, and lack of responsibility for owns health.

Therefore, being aware of this phenomenon, understanding and recognising it, make it possible for us to better understand our patients and act in a conscious way that would be in their favour.

8.4 Clinical Implications

Recognising and understanding the transference dynamics, projective identification, and regressive self-states in the medical encounter create a port of entry to our patients' psychic inner realm, and moreover protect us from potential relational ditches. By having a sense of understanding and experiencing our patients, we have the opportunity to get to know better their expectations, needs, and hopes. Our patients' hidden agenda would be more easily exposed and help us recognise some of their conscious and unconscious wishes and fears contributing to conflict or intense dependency (Hughes & Kerr, 2000). Furthermore, this kind of awareness at a subsequent meeting would enable us to be in a different state of mind, more receptive, mindful, and knowing, and less negative, angry, or hostile towards patients. This kind of presence and attitude cultivates rapport between doctor and patient, fosters a better communication, and is essential for good practice (Sklar, 2012). For instance, when meeting a patient like Jenny, who tends to be demanding, hostile, and angry, we might feel restless, anxious, and grumpy (which might be at least partially due to projective identification). These feelings reveal Jenny's inner experience and we can use this information to address her fears and wishes with less conflict and to better attend to her. Hence, we might take her behaviour less personally, be more empathic, and relate to her anxiety and fears more appropriately.

When we are aware of the transference towards us (the role that the patient grants us) and of regressive self-states we have more freedom regarding the role we take as doctors for our patients' beneficence. We might be more paternalistic or alternatively more enhancing patients' autonomy. For example, John comes helpless and anxious, unable to make medical decisions and take charge of his health (regressive self-state). We can take the role of the omnipotent, saving father and make decisions for him, or we can take a more mutual attitude enhancing collaboration with him in order to help him take charge of his illness and support him throughout the process (Funnell, 2000). Recognising his regressive self-state and the role he tries to enforce of us, helps us make a conscious choice rather than being drawn to complementary and reactive relationship.

Another example is a patient like Lisa, who is thankful and obedient, and idealises her doctor. While she might have appropriate affection mixed with idealisation, which contribute to her medical management and compliance, she could develop a wish for a more intimate relationship. If we are mindful of the transference dynamics, we can treat her with respect while being attentive to maintaining clear boundaries without humiliating her.

In this chapter we have tried to delve into the inner psychic experience of our patients by presenting you with the unconscious psychological phenomena of transference, projective identification, and regression that are common in the medical encounter. We believe that understanding of these processes enables doctors to grasp their patients' experience more deeply, get to know their hidden agenda, and react more thoughtfully rather than emotionally and unconsciously. Applying this knowledge in clinical practice is therapeutic for both patients and doctors. Patients' clinical management will be informed by a greater comprehension of their needs and motives, and doctors will be less vulnerable and overwhelmed by unrecognised projections.

Relationships are not a science; they are complicated lattice-like patterns which are often difficult, and sometimes impossible, to fully decipher. Getting a grip on transference dynamics can help us better understand why people behave as they do, and respond more humanly in the clinical situation, which is prone for strong emotional responses. To present a clear picture of transference dynamics, we have simplified complex patterns of behaviour, which form a significant part of the psychotherapist's training. Before moving on, we would like to just mention another complexity, and one which makes the doctor-patient relationship even more special and deserving of learning about. This complexity involves the doctor. While patients bring their history and past to their relationship with us, so do we carry our own habitual patterns of relating. We too often relate to our patients through the lenses of our past, we too transfer the ghosts of our past to the present time. This transference by the doctor is called countertransference, and will be looked at in the next chapter.

Together, transference and countertransference create a dance, which without recognition and understanding can frequently become a risky trap for the physician and the patient as well.

Note

1. This chapter contains revised paragraphs from *Touching the Relational Edge* (Rolef Ben-Shahar, 2014).

References

Fritzsche, K., Chen, F.K.Y., Jing, W., Frahm, G., & Monsalve, S.D. (2014). Balint group. In K. Fritzsche, S.H. McDaniel, & M. Wirsching (Eds.), *Psychosomatic medicine: An international primer for the primary care setting*. New York; Heidelberg; Dordrecht; London: Springer.

Funnell, M.M. (2000). Helping patients take charge of their chronic illnesses. *Family Practice Management, 7*(3), 47–51.

Hughes, P., & Kerr, I. (2000). Transference and countertransference in communication between doctor and patient. *Advances in Psychiatric Treatment-Journal of Continuing Professional Development, 6*, 57–64.

Rolef Ben-Shahar, A. (2014). *Touching the relational edge: Body psychotherapy*. London: Karnac Books.

Roter, D.L., & Hall, J.A. (2006). *Doctors talking with patients/patients talking with doctors: Improving communication in medical visits*. Westport, CT: Praeger Publishers.

Rothschild, B., & Rand, M.L. (2006). *Help for the helper: The psychophysiology of compassion fatigue and vicarious trauma*. New York, NY: W.W. Norton & Co.

Ryle, A. (1998). Transference and countertransference: The cognitive analytic perspective. *British Journal of Psychotherapy, 14*, 303–309.

Sklar, J. (2012). Regression and new beginnings: Michael, Alice and Enid Balint and the circulation of ideas. *Journal of International Psychoanalysis, 93*(4), 1017–1034.

Sullivan, H.S. (1954). Basic concepts in the psychiatric interview. *Pastoral Psychology, 5*(8).

9   The Doctor

Countertransference and
Narcissistic Traps

The ghosts of our past walk with our patients into our clinic room. Sometimes their attitudes towards us assist us in providing them with the healthcare they need. Sometimes these ghosts make our work that much harder. But
these ghosts walk with us just us well. We respond to our patients not solely
based on who they are and what they present us with but also, and oftentimes
much more so, based also on whom they remind us, on how we were accus-
tomed to respond and more. The way our past experiences influence the way
we perceive our patients and respond to them is called *countertransference*.
We both respond to one another based on our past patterns; transference and
countertransference are two sides to the same coin, together forming what is
known in psychotherapy as *transference-dynamics*. Psychoanalyst Hans Loewald (1986) wrote: "I believe it is ill-advised, indeed impossible, to treat transference and countertransference as separate issues. They are the two faces of
the same dynamic, rooted in the inextricable intertwining with others in which
individual life originates and remains throughout the life of the individual in
numberless elaborations, derivatives, and transformations" (p. 276).

Chapter 8 introduced the complexities, potentials, and risks involved in the
patients'-side of transference dynamics (transference), and this chapter will
elaborate on the physicians' side of this dynamics (countertransference).

*Maria, a 74-year-old woman suffering from rheumatoid arthritis, enters
your clinic accompanied by her daughter. Walking in with her cane, she sits
down in her chair, her face twitching with pain, when you notice her swollen
and deformed joints. You have known her for years. She is a rather polite and
quiet woman, and despite her compliance to all kinds of medical treatments
she keeps deteriorating. You have done everything you can, trying all kinds of
treatments, and consulting the best rheumatologists you could think of. When
you ask her about her symptoms and functionality, her daughter takes it upon
herself to answer your questions. "She is in pain, the pills recommended by the
rheumatologist have many side effects, and she can hardly sleep at night", she
answers readily.*

"And what do you say, Maria"? You ask her.

*Her eyes meet yours for a brief moment, when you hear her daughter
saying, "Well, you know doctor, I see her every day, she is not OK, nothing*

helps anymore, you have got to do something to help, she cannot go on like that".

> While reading this clinical example, how do you feel as Maria's doctor?
> What kinds of emotions are evoked in you towards Maria? Her daughter?
> How do you feel watching your patient's deterioration undeterred by medical treatments?
> How would you handle this situation?
> There is no right or wrong. Our interactions with patients, family members, and various clinical situations provoke in each of us myriad of feelings and reactions.

In this chapter, we will focus on the doctor's experience of these interactions; we will elaborate on the psychological phenomena of countertransference in the medical encounter, and address narcissistic traps in the doctor-patient relationship that might affect our feelings and responses.

9.1 Countertransference

The rigorous medical training and practice encompass acquiring vast clinical and theoretical knowledge together with communicative skills, entrusting doctors with the remarkable responsibility of treating patients. While there has been growing interest in the doctor-patient relationship in medical training, there are aspects of these challenging and complex interactions that can impede even the most experienced doctors (Moukkadam et al., 2016).

As demonstrated in the previous chapters, the doctor-patient relationship is an asymmetrical relationship, whereby the patient is in a passive and dependent position, compared to the doctor who carries his expertise. The medical encounter consists of mutual expectations and hopes, which may be conscious and explicit or may be unconscious, and therefore communicated in implicit ways (Balint, 1957; Hughes & Kerr, 2000). Moreover, we know that both patient and doctor bring along with them their professional and personal biographies to their encounter. These universal characteristics of the doctor-patient relationship make it prone to intricacy and complexity (Cosoli & Consoli, 2016).

Patients might reject our help, get angry and disappointed at us; they might touch our hearts; and they might revive our deepest wounds. Hence, over the course of our interactions with patients, we develop feelings which may affect the way we resolve and process our patients' problems. These feelings are sometimes responses to the patient's feelings and biographies (we call this *responsive countertransference*) and sometimes these are shadows of our own biographies we are responding to (*reactive countertransference*).

Since transference is an unavoidable psychological phenomenon that occurs in all relationships, as doctors we are affected too. We experience, consciously or unconsciously, a variety of emotions in each encounter with each particular patient. We respond to our patients' stories, age, gender, physical appearance, voice intonation, and character traits through the beliefs, generalisations, limitations, and distortions of our past relating (Consoli & Consoli, 2016; Rolef Ben-Shahar, 2014).

Countertransference is therefore the doctor's transference towards the patient. The countertransference response comprises of feelings, body sensations, and associated thoughts that could be activated as a response to the patient's transference, or emerge from the doctor's personal biography (Hughes & Kerr, 2000; Rolef Ben-Shahar, 2014). That means that we do not only respond unconsciously to our patients' life stories and transference communication, but also through the lenses of our own family, personal, and professional history.

Let us go back to the clinical example given above.

We might perceive Maria's daughter as intrusive and interfering, and our patient as a defenceless woman surrendering to her authoritative and overbearing daughter. Therefore, we might feel disturbed by the daughter's domineering attitude, and sorry for our patient. Alternately, we might perceive Maria's predilection as despicable and worthless, and her passive and inhibited demeanour might annoy us and make us angry. Obliviously we may continue our conversation with Maria's daughter, ignoring our patient, or we may interrupt abruptly her fluency and try to communicate with Maria.

On one hand, these emotional and behavioural responses are evoked by both Maria's and her daughter's transference communications, while each projects a different role on the doctor, eliciting different responses. On the other hand, each one of us will experience his own particular feelings, and respond in his own way in accordance to his own biographical lenses. That is to say that the degree to which the projected role (e.g., omnipotent father) adopted by the doctor, is congruent with the patient's conscious or unconscious wishes and is affected by the doctor's own elicited transferential patterns (Hughes & Kerr, 2000). The way each of us perceives Maria and her daughter would significantly impact our approach in the medical encounter. Both attitudes described above might weaken and jeopardise the therapeutic relationship with both of them, and have detrimental effect on clinical decisions.

The range of these aroused feelings in us can be very broad. It might extend from love to hatred, through sympathy, tenderness, sorrow, pity, irritation, exasperation, anger, disgust, confusion, despair, and rejection. While some of these feelings may be efficacious to the therapeutic alliance, others can entangle the doctor who experiences them without being aware of them. These "sentiment-traps" tend to hinder the doctor-patient relationship and bring forth inadequate attitudes in the doctor, which can conduct an erroneous assessment of the patient's medical condition, and affect medical treatment congruently (Cosoli & Consoli, 2016). Since countertransference is based on each individual's prior experiences and preconceived conceptions, each of us tends to be triggered by particular elements expressed in their patients. These triggers consist of various components such as gestures, intonations, certain behavioural patterns, and character traits which could have reminded us a significant person in our history (e.g., a dominant, controlling father). Some of us are activated by uncompliant patients; some are disposed to be highly triggered by boundary issues, while others tend to feel extremely threatened by mild aggressive behaviours. These kinds of transference dynamics may give rise to diverse reactions from aggressiveness, through rejection and pleasing behaviour. These kinds of reactions constitute the sequels of doctor acting out. It happens when we unconsciously play the role given to us by our patients and/or triggered by them in a way that provokes stress.

It is requisite to make a distinction between reacting and responding. A reaction is instant. It is driven by the beliefs, biases, and prejudices of the unconscious mind, and is survival-oriented. When we are trapped in transference dynamics and act through it, we react. The act of responding requires self-awareness of the circumstances, identification of the dynamics between us and our patient, and reflection. It is a conscious act. When we are entrapped in the transference dynamics without the capability of processing it, we might be trying to placate, deny, or rationalise, or we might project our feelings onto our patients (Timor, 2012). Being mindful and aware of our countertransference would enable us to respond rather than react.

When we are confronted with Maria's daughter dominating behaviour and Maria's passivity, our transferential patterns are activated and therefore we might react out of our anger, anxiety, despair, or helplessness. As a result, we can act aggressively and brusquely interrupt the daughter, or we can go forward our dialogue with her and exclude the mother. In contrast, we can take a pause and notice our immediate drive to react, realise that despite our irritation, both mother's and daughter's attitude are ensued by their suffering and is expressed in different ways. Then, we can avoid getting caught up in the transference dynamics and respond thoughtfully, rather than react emotionally.

9.2 Narcissistic Traps

Coming back from teaching a seminar in Europe, I am seated in my chair on a night flight, trying to sleep. Suddenly all the lights are turned on, a loud commotion. "Is there a doctor on the flight?" My heart is pounding. "He is having a heart attack", shouts the stewardess.

"Is there a doctor on the plane?"

Should I get up? Should I? I am not medically trained. Surely there is a doctor on the plane? But, I think, sometimes panic attacks resemble heart attacks. Perhaps this is psychological, in which case I could be of use; should I not check? Is it responsible to simply remain seated? But I always involve myself in these situations. I want to do something differently and remain seated. My mind is restless, though. I make a deal with myself: I will check if the man is attended to. If not I will get up. When the stewardess passes by I ask, "Did you find a doctor?" She nods.

In theory, now is the time to recline the chair and go back to sleep. However, I spend the remaining time of the flight struggling to let go of fact that I did not get up, and oscillating between being happy that I did not and feeling guilty for it.

I wonder if all the people on that night flight were as preoccupied with the question of getting up and providing some sort of help to this man. Would it have been different had the airplane been full of psychotherapists or doctors?

My supervisor said once that 90% of therapists, doctors, and healers have come to these professions to save their mothers. The remaining 10% are there to save their dads.[1]

In the courses and workshops we run, we often ask doctors about their motivations for choosing to implement their role in caring for patients. While responses vary according to each individual, we have observed that the caring vocation is oftentimes ingrained in a desire for sublime power over illness and death.

We all want to be good doctors. Medical training taught us to be perfect, never to fail, and to view our role as that of a saviour who cures others. From exigent training, through long hours and effort of residency, to intricate daily practice of medicine, we all have expectations. We wish to help patients get better; we want to be respected and valued by our patients as well as our colleagues. We spend time and resources for years of training in order to attain knowledge and skills, but also to bolster our self-confidence and maintain a stable self-worth.

What do we feel when being blamed and undervalued by our patients? What happens to us when we feel helpless by our inability to cure or save our patients?

Confronted with Maria's deterioration and her daughter's expectations from you, how do you feel? How do you feel when the professional role of the saviour who cures others dissipates and you find yourself with no weapons in the fight against deteriorating illness? What emotions arouse in you when patients and family members come with unrealistic expectations? What happens when feelings of inadequacy coexisting with your own expectations to be good doctors threaten your self-worth?

Narcissism is a complex concept which carries a variety of meanings, extending from a healthy and important developmental achievement to a potentially destructive personality disorder (Rolef Ben-Shahar, 2014). The foundation of healthy narcissism concerns agency—appropriately gauging our capacity to respond in this world. It is the feeling of self-esteem along with the ability to be self-confident and enjoy power in line with reality (Kohut, 1971). Narcissism is about being central agents in our own life and narcissistic injuries involve distorted perception of our power and centrality. It is not necessarily about feeling egotistical or self-important. In the airplane vignette, for instance, the feeling that the patient's suffering was my responsibility reflected a narcissistic position. Most people did not experience themselves activated by this man's pain, or responsible for helping him. We wish to emphasise, therefore, that a healthy amount of narcissism is not only necessary for a good life (someone who knows their worth and considers their desires and hopes to be important avenues to pursue), but is also important to make this world a better place—people who feel that they have to do something worthy manifest narcissistic tendencies. Pathological aspects of narcissism occur when the person either makes everything about them, for better or worse (if a patient's condition worsens, it is your personal responsibility and fault), or lose track of reality by being imbalanced in how they integrate responsibility with other factors.

Throughout life we have all experienced narcissistic injuries, when our self-worth has been threatened in our personal and professional life. Furthermore, we all have narcissistic wounds resulted by recurrent threats to our self-perception and due to deprivations of our own narcissistic needs. In her book *The Drama of the Gifted Child*, Alice Miller (1981) argues that many therapists (and we believe doctors too) share personality and biographical traits allowing them to be sensitive to others' needs, and enhance their need and motivation to give others, attempting to satisfy those deprivations and meeting those needs. Together with our genuine wish to help, we also search to nurture our own unmet needs, heal our subsequent narcissistic wounds, wishing to be emotionally rewarded by our patients and colleagues. We receive meaning and build the sense of our worth, when patients let us help them. When this need for gratitude and recognition is denied or disavowed by us as doctors, we run the risk of being captured by narcissistic traps.

Being trapped, we tend to interpret the situation through the lens of our "narcissistic-wound-glasses". We tend to be self-centred, asking ourselves what a certain difficulty says about us as doctors (Timor, 2012). We are going unconsciously through a self-evaluating process in which we perceive a particular incident in the medical encounter as jeopardising our self-image as good doctors, resulting in shame and a globalised negative view of ourselves (Tracy et al., 2011). In other words, we take it personally, and feel that it is all about us. We believe that learning about our motivation for becoming physicians is therefore of great value, and can help us discern (at least sometimes) what is ours and what is not.

Each one of us will be activated differently. We might feel a broad spectrum of feelings such as helplessness, guilt, shame, frustration, threat, or anger.

Each of us has his own strategies to deal with such narcissistic injuries, desperately trying to maintain a sense of self-worth.

We might be swept into narcissistic saving fantasies, believing we possess the power to save our patient (Epstein, 2016), and consequently endeavour to find more ways to treat our patient's chronic deteriorating illness in order to "save" her. We might seek to "get rid "of our patient; sometimes we will act defensively trying to prove our innocence; or we can find ourselves being aggressive or blaming our patients.

Being aware of our narcissistic needs and the narcissistic traps we are swamped in, is the first step needed for taking off our "narcissistic-wound-glasses". While doing so, we can reconnect with our genuine self-esteem and true wish to help patients as doctors, and allow ourselves to acknowledge our failures and limitations without defensiveness, anger, or shame. We will succumb less to the shame-destined attributable trap of blaming ourselves, and negative events might be attributed to specific actions. Nonetheless, hubristic pride in response to success will be replaced with authentic one emanated out of genuine self-esteem, unfolding feelings of confidence, productivity, and self-worth (Tracy et al., 2011). From an "it is all about me" point of view, we can broaden our apperception and see the other. We can look at Maria and her deterioration, feeling compassionate and accept with pain the limitations of medicine. We can perceive her daughter's demands as an expression of her anxiety and concern about her mother instead of blaming her.

9.3 Clinical Implications

As we have shown countertransference and narcissistic traps are part and parcel of our interactions with patients. Being caught unconsciously in transferential dynamics or in a narcissistic trap, we tend to react rather than respond. This might risk our clinical judgement, deviating us from beneficial professional behaviour, as well as endanger our well-being. One of the preponderant contributions of psychoanalysis to the understanding of the doctor-patient relationship is to have demonstrated the importance of being attuned not only to our patients, but also to ourselves, to our own feelings induced in the medical encounter (Consoli & Consoli, 2016).

Being aware of our feelings towards our patients, saviour fantasies, and narcissistic needs, recognising that we all have 'blind spots' and certain triggers that activate our own transferential patterns, are of paramount importance. When we are mindful to these psychological processes, and make the unconscious conscious, we can take a step back, and instead of being entrapped in a swirl of emotions, we can regulate ourselves (and our patients) and make better clinical choices.

When I notice my irritation and growing anger while encountering Maria and her daughter, I can take a brief pause and mindfully explore my sensations, emotions, and thoughts. I might feel tightness in my chest; I feel irritated by her controlling daughter, and angry about Maria's passive behaviour. I can also feel helpless and threatened by their expectations in view of my inability to fulfil them. I take a few seconds to regulate myself and connect with my resources (see chapter 5 and 6). Afterwards, I can breathe deeply and think more clearly. I can recognise my own biographical buttons being pressed, Maria's passivity reminds me of my father, and her daughter's domination resembles my mother's. I can also notice being trapped in my own narcissistic need for their recognition of all the efforts I have done for Maria for so many years.

Realising that I am hooked in these embroiled processes enables me get out of this emotional trap. Faced with Maria and her daughter, I can be sensitive and empathic to their suffering, listen to their request for assistance, and avoid acting impulsively or impatiently. I can listen to the daughter and accept her comments without invalidating them, while soliciting Maria's point of view whenever possible. Instead of feeling shameful due to my limitations and my cracked omnipotent self-perception leading to my trying to save her, and referring her to more unnecessary blood tests or specialist consultation, I can rather be present compassionately and empathically with her suffering and pain.

To conclude, being mindful and taking into account countertransference phenomena and narcissistic traps in the medical encounter can be applied as a useful clinical tool that can help us providing better medical care. When we have better understanding of these processes, we can be in a different state of mind that is clearer and more receptive. This will be therapeutic for both patient and doctor. The patient's clinical management will be less biased by unconscious emotions and behaviours; patient's needs and motives will be better addressed; and the doctor's better understanding and clarity will make him less vulnerable to being trapped emotionally.

Transference dynamics are among the most extensively explored themes in psychotherapy. Patients and therapists spend many years becoming more aware of how their past has influenced their present in order to free themselves, as much as possible, from reactions and allow for more conscious and informed responses. We wish to honour the work that is required in order to truthfully introspect and become aware of the forces that impact us in relationships, and reiterate that while some understandings could be gained alone, it might be very useful and transformative to go through this process with a professional psychotherapist.

Something to Think About

Who are the patients that mostly activate your transferential patterns? Do they remind you anyone from your past?

What kinds of triggers activate these patterns? Certain character traits? Gestures? Words?

If you could save anybody, who would you have saved?

Note

1. A previous version of this vignette was taken from my chapter in *When Hurt Remains* (Rolef Ben-Shahar, 2016).

References

Balint, M. (1957). *The doctor, his patient and the illness*. London: Pitman.

Consoli, S.G., & Consoli, S.M. (2016). Countertransference in dermatology. *Acta Dermato-Venereologica, 217*, 18–21.

Epstein, S. (2016). Failing with dignity. In A. Rolef Ben-Shahar & R. Shalit (Eds.), *When hurt remains: Relational perspectives on therapeutic failure* (pp. 79–86). London: Karnac Books.

Hughes, P., & Kerr, I. (2000). Transference and countertransference in communication between doctor and patient. *Advances in Psychiatric Treatment-Journal of Continuing Professional Development, 6*, 57–64.

Kohut, H. (1971). *The analysis of the self: A systematic approach to the psychoanalytic treatment of narcissistic personality disorders*. Madison, CT: International Universities Press.

Loewald, H.W. (1986). Transference-countertransference. *Journal of the American Psychoanalytic Association, 34*, 275–287.

Miller, A. (1981). *The drama of the gifted child*. New York, NY: Basic Books.

Moukkadam, N., Tucci, V., Galwankar, S., & Shah, A. (2016). In the blink of an eye: Instant countertransference and its application in modern healthcare. *Journal of Emergency Trauma Shock, 9*, 95–96.

Rolef Ben-Shahar, A. (2014). *Touching the relational edge: Body psychotherapy*. London: Karnac Books.

Rolef Ben-Shahar, A. (2016). Losing my religion? Psychotherapeutic practices repetition compulsion of character rigidity. In A. Rolef Ben-Shahar & R. Shalit (Eds.), *When hurt remains: Relational perspectives on therapeutic failure* (pp. 149–156). London: Karnac Books.

Timor, G. (2012). Humanizing perfectionism: A journey of a client and a beginning body-psychotherapist. *British Journal of Psychotherapy Integration, 9*(1), 7–16.

Tracy, J.L., Cheng, J.T., Martens, J.P., & Rolef, R.W. (2011). The emotional dynamics of narcissism: Inflated by pride, deflated by shame. In W.K. Campbell & J.D. Miller (Eds.), *The handbook of narcissism and narcissistic disorder: Theoretical approaches, empirical findings, and treatments* (pp. 330–343). Hoboken, NJ: Wiley.

10 Tenets of Human Presence, Empathy, and Compassion

> How do you expect to make your living except by meeting your patients, by respecting and liking them—by thoroughly liking them? You ought not to have any other attitude toward patients than one of sympathy and liking and respect.
> —Milton Erickson (1965, p. 272)

We are in the middle of patient rounds, passing by numerous patients, talking to them and their relatives, examining them thoroughly, looking at their laboratory test results, discussing intricate cases, and brainstorming various clinical solutions. I am totally concentrated on the tasks I have to fill during my shift, when I find us standing by an eighty-nine-year-old woman with Alzheimer and pneumonia. I am impatient, briefly looking at her vital signs and her chest X-ray, assuring an appropriate antibiotic, and finding myself ready to move on to the next patient. We are all moving forward, when I see him, one of our residents, approaching her gently, putting his hand on her shoulder while softly saying: "Good morning, Ruth, how are you?"

I slow down, my impatience and rushing attitude fades, a vibrating feeling fills my heart reminding me the quality of humanity. Tenderness and softness arise in me. My entire presence is affected by this precious moment; I can look at Ruth and see a human being, someone who was once a child, a teenager, a lover, a wife, a mother, and a grandmother. Someone who could have been my grandmother, my mother, me. How easily I forget. Her eyes are closed and her body is still. It has been long time since she could talk, no noticeable reaction except for one long deep breath, and a significant lesson in human presence, empathy, and compassion for me.

Ruth is one of those patients whom we cannot cure. How easily we are drawn to a technical, skilful, rational, and emotionally detached attitude, over-valuing scientific measures and disconnecting from our humanity. These kinds of encounters confront us with the unavoidable tension in the physician's role. On one hand, we strive for professionalism and detachment in order to make appropriate clinical decisions, while on the other hand, we endeavour to reconnect a compassionate attitude, honouring our patients, acknowledging suffering, and expressing respect and warmth towards them. Various guidelines and recommendations highlighting the importance of empathy, compassion, and human presence as fundamental requirements of medical care have been published in recent years (Epstein, 2017; Kerasidou & Horn, 2016). However, in practice doctors find it challenging to interlace technical skills and these human values which demand emotional engagement. Concerns regarding increasingly dehumanisation of medical practice has been raised (Haslam, 2006).

In this chapter we portray the significance of human presence, empathy, and compassion in medical care, we discuss their influence on both patients and doctors, we examine the intricacies and obstacles in applying them in medicine, and we represent ways to cultivate those qualities for our own benefit as well as our patients'.

10.1 Human Presence

Encountering Ruth, I found it difficult to look at the humanity of a woman with long-standing, deteriorating Alzheimer's disease and acute pneumonia. Reflexively, I endorse my gaze in order to refrain from expressions of pain and suffering, and engage with my tasks. Our resident's quality of being, expressed in a few gentle words and a simple gesture, represents human presence in medical care.

Human presence is a quality of being, and it describes a therapeutic stance and positioning more than a therapeutic skill or act. It necessitates us to be open to human connection, to be present to ourselves, and to be willing to assume responsibility for our feelings, capacities, and limitations with acceptance (Totton, 2003). There is no wonder that for many physicians this is a near-impossibility. We join medical school as young adults, frequently incapable of withstanding the deep emotional complexities that accompany human conditions, even if our minds are at their sharpest to absorb medical information. Human presence therefore needs to be cultivated, gently and humbly. It is a quality of listening without judging, interpreting, or interrupting. Its foundation is in a feeling of bonding between two people that are attuned to each other. It comprises the sense of dignity and respect when patients need it most (Epstein, 2017; Rolef Ben-Shahar, 2014). Being present encompasses reconnecting with our innate virtue of loving and dignifying humanity, deeply accepting pain and suffering as an integral part of life, and staying with hurtful experiences without fighting, escaping, or dissociating. It might be communicated verbally, but more often it is communicated non-verbally by a soft look at the patient's eyes, a gentle quality of touch, and a respectful way of physical examination; it is our willingness to drop our white coat and be human, while at the same time maintain our professional knowledge and responsibility. It is about doctors being able to see each patient as a human being.

Human presence awards patients with the feeling of being understood, cared for, honoured, and respected by their doctor. Therefore, it is a vital quality for health care, and is the basis of trust and a precondition for offering a therapeutic relationship (Epstein, 2017; Totton, 2003). On the ground of human presence in medical care the seeds of empathy and compassion can sprout and thrive.

10.2 Empathy

Empathy can be defined in many ways. It is often described as the capacity to experience another's perspectives and feelings. It is an introspective process in which the doctor attempts to find in him a similar experience to that of the patient. In other words, empathy entails sensing what it is like to be our patient (Haslam, 2006; Kohut, 1982). This process engages a transition from an intra-psychic experience (our experiences are internally felt as separate individuals) to an interpersonal one (our experiences are dialectically felt in the relational field—a lattice of interconnected influences) which is based on cognitive, affective, and bodily domains. The cognitive aspect of empathy refers to the comprehension of the experience from the patient's point of view (*I can see how it might feel if I were you*). For example, when a patient is diagnosed with new diabetes mellitus, we understand that it is difficult for him. The affective element relates to the ability to feel the other emotionally (*I hurt when I think of you, when I feel how it might feel to be you*). That is to say, that together with understanding the experience, we can feel the patient's helplessness and frustration within us. The bodily domain refers to the ability to bodily sense the patient's experience (*I can sense in my body what it is like to be you*). Meaning that I understand my patient's distress, I can feel it emotionally, and I can sense my breath a little heavier and a lump in my throat (Epstein, 2017; Kerasidou & Horn, 2016).

When we witness our patients' pain and suffering, bodily empathy is immediate and tangible. Whether we acknowledge it or not, whether we wish for it or not, our body converses with the other person's body, directly and without conscious mediation. If we are mindful, we can observe that we might feel our patient's pain in our own body, and imitate her facial expression or bodily posture. The neurobiologist Damasio (1994, 2003) terms the phenomenon of direct body communication "somatic markers theory" and proposes that emotional experiences begin with a physiological process of the body. This process constitutes the foundation of shared experience and affective resonance which is the route to understanding both emotions and bodily experiences, even when we have not had these specific experiences ourselves (Rudebeck, 2000). We can hear an echo of this bewildering process in Freud's (1915) own words: "It is a very remarkable thing that the unconscious can react upon another, without passing through consciousness" (p. 126).

The discovery of mirror neurons in 1990s (Gallese et al., 1996) has led to a cross-disciplinary revolution in the study of empathy. Mirror neurons belong to a specialised group of neurons located in the premotor cortex and the inferior parietal cortex. When we observe other people's activities, these neurons are activated and our brains stimulate what it is like to engage in that action. Some scientists have surmised that some areas in the brain, like the anterior cingulate cortex, interpret not only physical actions but also their associated emotional affect. Furthermore, studies indicate that for a motor neuron to be activated, we need to be affectively activated by observing the other (Gallese et al., 2002; Lamm & Singer, 2010; Reiss, 2010). In other words, being emotionally touched necessitates resonance; when we observe our patients' pain and suffering, it needs to be affectively meaningful for us, to activate bodily resonance. These emotional bodily resonance systems are the basis of emotional intelligence, and allow us to feel the other through our own bodies by breaking the walls between us (Epstein, 2017). Research shows that while humans (doctors included) share neuroanatomical representations of pain, they experience the other's pain in an attenuated form. That is to say the observer has the capability to experience the other's pain to the extent that cultivates an empathic response without overwhelming the observer (Lamm et al., 2007; Singer & Lamm, 2009).

Therefore, empathy embraces a nonverbal attunement to patients' emotional and bodily cues, that fosters the possibility to recognise what it feels like to experience something, and to sense emotional connection and caring without being over identified. It is important to point out that the phenomenon of resonance has bi-directional effect. While we are affected by our patients' distress and pain, our patients are affected by our emotional state. That is why empathy is the basis for human connection in general and in medical care in particular. The early attempts of psychoanalysis to filter out the influence of the analyst, and the gradual understanding that such an act is impossible (Mitchell, 2005), further amplifies the need to attend to our own feelings and ensure we take our well-being with utmost care. Empathy and the physiological structures that enable it, are a central skill and character trait essential for a mutual engagement of doctor and patient, enabling us to translate our humanity, demonstrate it, and act compassionately (Hadad & Rolef Ben-Shahar, 2012; Svenaeus, 2014). Halpern (2014) alleges that being empathic means neither being nice nor avoiding feeling negative feelings towards patients. She stresses that empathy is about seeing, understanding, and caring for patients, and granting them with the feeling of being seen, perhaps not unlike the quote from Milton Erickson at the beginning of this chapter.

There is a large body of research emphasising the positive effects of empathy on patient care. Empathy has been related to better communication, increased patients' participation, satisfaction, and compliance, decreased emotional distress, enhanced therapeutic efficacy, and positive physiologic effects that improve outcomes (Halpern, 2003; Larson & Yao, 2005; Mercer & Reynolds, 2002; Neumann, 2011; Reiss, 2010). In recent years, medical literature has given more attention to the impact of empathy on doctors and their well-being. Evidence suggests that empathy makes practicing medicine more meaningful, enriches the experiencing of doctoring, and therefore decreases symptoms of burnout (Halpern, 2003; Reiss, 2010). Looking at it from a psychotherapeutic perspective, we can say that it is harder (and more stress-provoking) to invest our energy in rejecting the other person's experiences than it is to allow this natural influence to take space.

So how come implementing empathy in medical practice is arduous? Why is it so hard to see Maria as a human being? Why is it so complicated to engage empathically with our patients' pain, frustration, anger, non-compliance, etc.?

How can we explain the decreasing empathy along the years of practicing medicine?

There is now considerable growing evidence demonstrating significant declines in empathy in medical school, residency, and beyond (Bellini & Shea, 2005; Haslam, 2006; Neunann, 2011). This decline has been attributed to various factors: low sense of well-being, emotional distress, self-protective disengagement from patients' suffering, sense of hopelessness in the confronting therapeutic failure, over identification with patients, growing reliance on technology, and economic and time constraints by health care systems (Bellini et al., 2002; Haslam, 2006; Neunann, 2011; Stratton et al., 2008; Shanafelt et al., 2005; Thomas et al., 2007).

All these factors point to a painful conclusion: practicing medicine is dangerous for our well-being as physicians. We have proposed in this book that addressing difficulties rather than repressing them is conductive to our health and well-being as practitioners. As we can see, the most influencing factor is emotional distress caused by encountering unavoidable pain and suffering in medical care. While mirror neuron activity is linked to empathic function, it seems that anxiety, stress, and tension can significantly reduce the signal rate of mirror neurons diminishing the ability to empathise. Moreover, in a neuroimaging controlled study observing doctors response to others pain, physicians down-regulated their pain empathy response by inhibiting neural circuits involved in pain processing areas (Decety et al., 2010). We conclude that constant exposure to pain and suffering and the unavoidable result of personal emotional distress have physiologic effects on our ability to empathise.

These findings have revived a long history of discussion and debate regarding the possible significance of clinical detachment in medical care. As already shown, empathy in medical care has a large number of benefits for both patients and doctors. In contrast, some researchers plead that being genuinely empathic with patients might be emotionally draining and intricate under modern time constraints. They argue that by not becoming emotionally involved with patients, the detached doctor is capable of making objective decisions concerning their care (Halpern, 2012; Zinn, 1993). Several arguments have been made in favour of doctor emotional detachment. Physicians learn to prosper emotional detachment in order to preserve their medical objectivity in distressing situation, avoiding strong emotional involvement and over-identification with their patients (Lief & Fox, 1963). Moreover, some researchers support the idea that doctors need to sustain an emotional detachment in order to shield them from distress and manage their emotions (Sanchez-Reilly et al., 2013; Sokol, 2012; Stanton & Noble, 2010).

Might clinical detachment be a good solution for preserving our well-being as doctors?

In Part I we have shown how trying to refrain from engaging emotionally with our patients can seriously impact on our health and psychological well-being (see chapters 2 and 3). In a study investigating the way physician dispositions relate to behavioural measures of pain sensitivity, empathy, and professional well-being, the researchers found that professional experience desensitise physicians to pain of others without helping them down-regulate their own personal distress (Gleichgerrcht & Decety, 2014). Epstein (2017) addresses the paradox of empathy. He shares with the readers how he has surveyed students and residents and found that some of those who score highest on empathy are sometimes the most burned out. He honestly asks if too much empathy in medicine might be toxic. He reckons that while we have been training students and doctors to share emotions and take the patient's perspective, we have failed in helping them cultivate self-awareness and manage their strong feelings. The absence of these two essential elements might cause doctors to feel traumatised, making them disconnect and adopt a cool objective stance. Epstein finds the solution in training physicians to be compassionate not only for the sake of their patients, but also as an antidote to emotional tension and burnout. We would like to further argue that implementing a doctor-centred attitude in medicine as presented in chapter 4 is a prerequisite for cultivating an empathic stance in medicine. As we have been shown, emotional distress is a major cause of diminishing clinical empathy. Therefore, we believe that applying regularly self-care practices, developing and connecting to a variety of resources, and developing mindful self-awareness, as elaborated in chapter 5 and 6, have the potential to make the endowment of empathic practice possible.

As a last thought on empathy, we wish to discuss habit formation. Our human ability to form habitual structures is uncanny. Our autopilot modes free us to engage with multiple requirements. By spending most of our working hours actively trying to detach our emotions, we cultivate a habit of detaching. It is hard to reconnect emotionally in our personal lives, with our loved ones, when we have become so practiced in checking out.

Is this really the life we ask for ourselves?

10.3 Compassion

Compassion is defined as the ability "to suffer with" (Haq, 2014) and incorporates three major elements (Epstein, 2017). The first two elements comprise of (1) noticing another's suffering and (2) resonating with it—that is, feeling the other person both from the outside, and from within. As we have already delineated in the previous section these two components define empathy. The third element of compassion is (3) taking action with intention to alleviate suffering. Is it not the physician's creed? Being compassionate means recognising and acknowledging suffering, expressing empathy, respect, and warmth, honouring patients' needs and wishes, and supporting them and their families.

Studies show that compassion engenders trust in the doctor-patient relationship, decreases the burden of patients' suffering, and helps them heal (Epstein, 1999; Siegel, 2012). Furthermore, it appears that compassionate practice nourishes doctors with an enhanced sense of purpose, well-being, affiliation, and belonging deriving from physiologic effects such as release of endogenous opioids, dopamine and oxytocin (Klimecki, 2014).

While realising the benefits of compassion in medicine, we are curious about its scarceness in daily practice. Compassionate practice requires ongoing commitment to our mission as doctors, not merely our daily tasks.

Epstein (2017) attempts to answer this question. He assumes that the answer rests in the second ingredient of compassion which is resonance with the other's suffering. He describes a series of experiments in which participants who were trained to resonate with others suffering without being given skills of translating it into compassion, were more emotionally distressed and activated in areas of brain known to be related to anxiety and distress. After a short practice aimed to conjure up compassion, these same people's brain scans showed that their "reward pathways" were activated instead of the distress ones. Hence, we conclude that physician should be given tools to cultivate compassion. Such tools are harder to learn, and even more to implement, when we are young people fully committed to learning the basics of anatomy, physiology, and pathology, young people who may be taught to view the emotional and relational component of medicine is a secondary necessity.

As we can see, human presence, empathy, and compassion are all interconnected, and each component affects the other. While these elements comprise a crucial part in the practice of medicine, we have demonstrated and depicted the intricacies and obstacles in implementing them in practice.

In the next chapter we hope to present practical ways to implement and apply those essential elements in daily practice based on research and our own experience.

References

Bellini, L.M., Baime, M., & Shea, J.A. (2002). Variation of mood and empathy during internship. *Journal of American Medical Association, 287*, 3143–3146.

Bellini, L., & Shea, J. (2005). Mood change and empathy decline persist during three years of internal medicine training. *Academic Medicine, 80*, 164–167.

Damasio, A. (1994). *Descartes' error: Emotion, reason, and the human brain.* New York, NY: Penguin Group.

Damasio, A. (2003). *Looking for Spinoza: Joy, sorrow and the feeling brain.* New York; London: Harcourt.

Daum, H., & Hartman, A. (2010). *Mind the road* (Hebrew ed.). Tel Aviv, Israel: Yediot Aharonot, Sifre Hemed.

Decety, J., Yang, C.Y., & Cheng, Y. (2010). Physicians down-regulate their pain empathy response: An event- related brain potential study. Neuroimage, 50(4), 1676–1682.

Epstein, R.M. (1999). Mindful practice. *Journal of American Medical Association, 282*(9), 833–839.

Epstein, R.M. (2017). *Attending: Medicine, mindfulness and humanity*. New York, NY: Scribner.

Erickson, M.H. (1965). An introduction to the study and the application of hypnosis in pain control. In E.L. Rossi, M.O. Ryan, & F.A. Sharp (Eds.), *The seminars, workshops and lectures of Milton H. Erickson: Vol. I: Healing in hypnosis* (pp. 217–277). London: Free Association Books, 1992.

Freud, S. (1915). The unconscious. *S. E., 14*, 159–215. London: Hogarth, 1957.

Gallese, V., Fadiga, L., Fogassi, L., & Rizzolatti, G. (1996). Action recognition in the premotor cortex. *Brain, 119*, 593–609.

Gallese, V., Ferrari, P.F., & Umita, M.A. (2002). The mirror matching system: A shred manifold for intersubjectivity. *Behavioral and Brain Sciences, 25*(1), 35–36.

Gleichgerrcht, E., & Decety, J. (2014). The relationship between different facets of empathy, pain perception and compassion fatigue among physicians. *Frontiers in Behavioral Neuroscience, 8*(243), 1–9.

Hadad, E., & Rolef Ben-Shahar, A. (2012). The things we're taking home with us: Understanding therapist's self-care in trauma work. *International Journal of Psychotherapy, 16*(1), 50–61.

Halpern, J. (2003). What is clinical empathy? *Journal of General Internal Medicine, 18*(8), 670–674.

Halpern, J. (2012). Attending to clinical wisdom. *Journal of Clinical Ethics, 23*(1), 41–46.

Halpern, J. (2014). From idealized clinical empathy to empathic communication in medical care. *Medicine, Health Care and Philosophy, 17*(2), 301–311.

Haq, C. (2014). Compassion in medicine. *Family Medicine, 46*(7), 549–550.

Haslam, N. (2006). Dehumanization: An integrative review. *Personality and Social Psychology Review, 10*, 252–264.

Kerasidou, A., & Horn, R. (2016). Making space for empathy: Supporting doctors in the emotional labour of clinical care. *BMC Medical Ethics, 17*(8).

Klimecki, O.M. (2014). Differential pattern of functional brain plasticity after compassion and empathy training. *Social Cognitive and Affective Neuroscience, 9*(6), 873–879.

Kohut, H. (1982). Introspection, empathy, and the semi-circle of mental health. *International Journal of Psychoanalysis, 63*, 395–407.

Lamm, C., Nusbaum, H.C., Meltzoff, A.N., & Decety, J. (2007). What are you feeling? Using functional magnetic resonance imaging to assess the modulation of sensory and affective responses during empathy for pain. *PLoS ONE, 12*, e1292.

Lamm, C., & Singer, T. (2010). The role of anterior insular cortex in social emotions. *Brain Structure and Function, 214*, 579–591.

Larson, E.B., & Yao, Y. (2005). Clinical empathy as emotional labor in the patient-physician relationship. *Journal of American Medical Association, 293*, 1100–1106.

Lief, H.I., & Fox, R.C. (1963). Training for "detached concern" in medical students. *Psychological Basis of Medical Practice, 12*, 35.

Mercer, S.W., & Reynolds, W.J. (2002). Empathy and quality of care. *British Journal of General Practice, 52*(supplement), S9-S13.

Mitchell, S.A. (2005). *Influence and autonomy in psychoanalysis*. Hillsdale, NJ: Analytic Press.

Neumann, M. (2011). Empathy decline and its reasons: A systematic review of studies with medical students and residents. *Academic Medicine, 86*(8), 996–997.

Reiss, H. (2010). Empathy in medicine a neurobiological perspective. *JAMA, 304*(14), 1604–1605.

Rolef Ben-Shahar, A. (2014). *Touching the relational edge: Body psychotherapy.* London: Karnac Books.

Rudebeck, C.E. (2000). The doctor, the patient and the body. *Scandinavian Journal of Primary Health Care, 18*(1), 4–8.

Sanchez-Reilly, S., Morrison, L.J., Carey, E., Bernacki, R., O'Neil, L., Kapo, J., et al. (2013). Caring for oneself to care for other: Physicians and their self- care. *Journal of Supportive Oncology, 11*(2), 75.

Shanafelt, T.D., West, C., Zhao, X., et al. (2005). Relationship between increased personal well-being and enhanced empathy among internal medicine resident. *Journal of General Internal Medicine, 20*(7), 559–564.

Siegel, D.J. (2012). *The developing mind, second edition: How relationships and the brain interact to shape who we are.* New York, NY: Guilford Press.

Singer, T., & Lamm, C. (2009). The social neuroscience of empathy. *Annals of NY Academy Science, 1156*, 81–96.

Sokol, D.K. (2012). How to be a cool headed clinician. *British Medical Journal, 344*, e3980.

Stanton, E., & Noble, D. (2010). Emotional intelligence. *BMJ Careers.*

Stratton, T.D., Saunders, J.A., & Elam, C.L. (2008). Changes in medical students' emotional intelligence: An exploratory study. *Teaching and Learning Medicine, 20*, 279–284.

Svenaeus, F. (2014). The phenomenology of empathy in medicine: An introduction. *Medical Health and Philosophy, 17*(2), 245–248.

Thomas, M.R., Dyrbye, L.N., Huntington, J.L., et al. (2007). How do distress and well-being relate to medical student empathy? A multicenter study. *Journal of General Internal Medicine, 22*, 177–183.

Totton, N. (2003). *Body psychotherapy: An introduction.* Maidenhead, UK: Open University Press.

Zinn, W. (1993). The empathic physician. *Archives of Internal Medicine, 153*, 306–312.

11 Just Be There

Implementing Human Presence, Empathy, and Compassion in Clinical Practice

I was practicing family medicine in a small town, where a great part of my patients came from a low socioeconomic class including unemployed people, former prisoners, and drug users. I was faced with quite a lot of aggressiveness and verbal violence. When I saw some of the specific names of those patients on my list, my whole body contracted, I got emotionally disconnected and impatient even before they came in. Let this day be over. I remember feeling frustrated, impatient, unsatisfied, and unable to find empathy and compassion in myself. Practicing medicine turned into technical, rational, and emotional detached. Doctoring became disconnected from humanity and hence meaningless.

One day I decided to conduct a little experiment and call for some of my difficult patients for an annual check-up, with an intention of listening to their life story with genuine curiosity and open heart. Most of them acceded to my call and came to the clinic. Before meeting each of them, I took a few moments to resource myself and attune myself to empathy and compassion. Despite my intention and a thread of hope, I was quite sceptical regarding the results. Listening to their stories with no judgement, adopting an empathic and compassionate attitude, although not without difficulties, turned to be one of the most powerful experiences I have had as a doctor. It was like a magic converting aggressiveness into sorrow and violence into helplessness. The rough and pugnacious man became the beaten child fighting to survive, and the tough former prisoner became the little boy taking care of his sick mother, robbing people in order to buy his mother's medications. I was astounded by the powerful impact it had on me as a doctor. My heart was open; humanity came into practice again engendering satisfaction and meaningfulness. However, the magic did not last, and I have learnt that cultivating human presence, empathy, and compassion needs regular practice. I believe it worth it.

In the previous chapter we have introduced the qualities of human presence, empathy, and compassion in medical care, elaborating on their beneficial effects for both patients and doctors, and discussed the difficulties in implementing them in clinical practice. Albeit the well-known positive affect these qualities have on therapeutic outcomes, doctors receive little or no formal training in cultivating these essential and influential therapeutic skills.

Medical literature suggests that it is possible to teach doctors these qualities (DasGupta & Charon, 2004; Platt & Keller, 1994; Reiss, 2010; Taigman, 1996). Though these qualities differ somewhat in their meanings, they all share the essence of kindness. A therapeutic attitude based on kindness and regular practice constitutes the foundation for culminating in these qualities.

In this chapter we will present practical ways for implementing human presence, empathy, and compassion in daily practice, integrating theory, our experience, and exercises for regular practice. We wish to emphasise that all the practices mentioned here are skills, and thus require cultivation. Without practice, it would be hard to utilise them successfully.

11.1 Resourcing

As shown in the previous chapter, one of the major obstacles for human presence, empathy, and compassion is emotional distress. In order to be fully present, to connect with our humanity, and attune in an empathic and compassionate attitude to our patients, we need to feel safe and calm by fostering our well-being. Self-regulation strategies alleviate emotional distress and are beneficial in intricate situations. In the example given in the beginning of this chapter, I used resourcing practices before encountering these challenging patients.

In chapter 5, we have introduced the magnitude of regularly applying self-care practices that cultivate well-being and enable the formation of healthier coping strategies. We have exemplified practical skills of self-care and a variety of resources to connect to, such as: centring, grounding, and breathing exercises. We believe that these practices are prerequisite for fostering human presence, empathy, and compassion in medical care. These exercises can be used on a regular basis as well as in intricate and intractable moments. Starting the day with five to ten minutes of practicing these exercises could make a significant change in the way we feel and meet our patients.

11.2 Intention

Deciding to conduct my little experiment and call for some of my difficult patients, I had a clear intention. Out of my frustration, I wished to listen to my patients' life stories with genuine curiosity and open heart so I could reconnect with my humanity and kindness. While being kind, fully present, empathic, and compassionate is a way of being, it calls for intention in order to emerge and thrive. Intention endows us with direction to our endeavours and refuels us with motivation.

Sometimes, intention to be kind, empathic, and compassionate is a practice of itself.

Sit quietly, and ask yourself honestly, how willing you are to enrich your practice with these qualities?

Try to imagine yourself abundant with empathy and compassion in your practice, and notice mindfully how it feels.

It might be interesting to do so also with imagining the same qualities in your personal life.

Be aware of your body sensations, feelings, and thoughts.

It might feel pleasant, or it might rise up fears or resistance.

Be curious about your intention.

11.3 I Am Here: Cultivating Human Presence in Medical Care

Consider this question—how do you meet your patients? Not what you do, what you know, nor what you say or even think. How do you meet your patients? What parts of you as a human being arrive to meet the other human being who happens to be your patient?

Human presence is a quality of being and it represents a therapeutic approach rather than a therapeutic skill or act. It refers to a unique individual combination of several elements, laying on the foundation of mindfulness. Each element needs to be present in balance with the other (Morgan & Morgan, 2005). To be fully present, we need to pay attention to our feelings, thoughts, and bodily sensations, and they need to be accessible to us (Stern, 2004). In addition to this mindful being we need to cultivate tranquillity, clarity of mind, curiosity, genuine interest in our patients, and the quality of deep listening to them. As already discussed in previous chapters, connecting to resources and practicing mindfulness, nurture clarity and tranquillity. Natural curiosity and genuine interest about our patients' lives are essential for fostering human presence and empathic stance. Being trained to take rapid, standardised histories, doctors learn to subdue curiosity in medical practice (Halpern, 2003). Curiosity can be cultivated by encouraging doctors to listen to patients' first-person story of illness and then tell or write narrative histories (Coles, 1989; Charon, 2001). Curiosity and genuine interest are necessary for deep listening. For which we need to be attentive, curious, interested in the other, be aware of our impulses to interpret, judge, or criticise, and deliberately put them aside for the time being. Doctors undergo a rigorous training in asking questions and looking for answers, that is—diagnosing and intervening. The practice of curiosity can therefore feel somewhat foreign—remaining curious (asking) without seeking answers (solutions).

As we can see, practicing mindfulness is the part and parcel of human presence, nurturing each element mentioned. In chapter 5, we have described an exercise for practicing mindfulness. This simple exercise practiced with centring, grounding, and breathing exercises offer some simple but deep ways to cultivate human presence in daily practice.

11.4 I See You: Implementing Empathy in Medical Care

While teaching doctors communicating skills, I often ask doctors to play their "difficult" patient in a role play. Before we start the experience, I instruct the doctor to adopt his patient's posture, speech, and way of being. I also advise him to imagine that he is his own patient with the specific illness, pains, difficulties, family status, and feelings, sitting there in front of his doctor. Following these instructions, we start the role play. Getting into their patients' shoes, most doctors experience a significant transformation in their attitude to their "difficult" patient.

The ability to experience someone else's way of being, feelings, and perspectives is the foundation of empathy. When we are attuned to feel our patient, intend and endeavour to sense his private world as seen and experienced as if it were our own without losing the "as if" quality, we are empathic. Occasionally, empathy is natural and effortless, and at other times we find it inaccessible. Our capacity for empathy fluctuates from day to day and moment to moment and depends on professional and personal variables. We can summon empathy in different ways. One of the crucial steps is feeling safe and relaxed together with an intention and openness to let ourselves go into our patients with acceptance and willingness. Afterwards, we may try to actively deepen our understanding of our patients' experience by letting ourselves resonate with them, deepening our listening, including psychosocial history in anamnesis, paying attention to transferential processes and narcissistic traps (see chapters 8 and 9), and imagining ourselves or our relatives in a similar situation. All of these elements demand self-awareness of our own sensations, emotions, and thoughts. Being empathic means that I experience the other's pain in me. The capacity of feeling the other's pain and suffering, on one the hand, while seeing them as distinct from our own, on the other hand (without being "caught emotionally"), is crucial (Halpern, 2001). Even though some of us are naturally more empathetic, without cultivating and prioritising these skills, we would lose our attunement or over-identify with the other.

How can it be done? After developing skills for cultivating empathy, how can we refrain from being "emotionally caught" without losing our presence?

In the previous chapter, we have mentioned a series of experiments in which participants who were trained to resonate with others suffering without being given skills of translating it into compassion, were more emotionally distressed and activated in areas of brain known to be related to anxiety and distress, consequently less capable of being present and express an empathic and compassionate attitude. Empathy requires that we be interested, willing, and capable of revisiting or experiencing a painful event and its corresponding affect.

There are some ways that might help us remain fully present while experiencing the other's pain. Resourcing and practicing mindfulness, as already mentioned, cultivate human presence and empathy. Compassion training, as will be discussed in the next section, has a major contribution too.

Another aspect is taken from Buddhist psychology and is based on a deep understanding of impermanence and suffering in life (Morgan & Morgan, 2005). From this viewpoint, while pain should be accepted as an integral and unavoidable part of life, misperceiving this nature of life, grasping illusions, and avoiding feeling pain, create and amplify suffering. In other words, when we encounter our patients' pain (as well as ours), staying with our feelings, understanding and accepting the impermanent nature of life, without fighting it or avoiding it, might alleviate our suffering. It does not mean that as doctors we do not make efforts to cure and save people, but it does mean that we accept this nature of life, without running away, abandoning our patients (and ourselves), or fighting the unavoidable nature of life. Human presence, empathy, and compassion are the natural offspring of this understanding, which is cultivated by practicing mindfulness.

11.5 I Am Here With You: Implementing Compassion in Medical Care

In chapter 5, we have addressed self-compassion as an active practice for cultivating kindness and caring towards oneself in the face of personal inadequacies, mistakes, failures, painful life situations, and suffering. We have noted that kindness and mindfulness are fundamental elements of self-compassion that encompasses self-kindness and understanding toward ourselves rather than judgement and self-criticism, perceiving our own experiences as part of humanity rather than as separating and isolating; and being mindfully aware of painful thoughts and feelings rather than over-identifying with them. We exemplified how self-compassion could be applied in medical care, and highlighted its rewards. This is a dynamic balance—it will change throughout our lives, we cannot reach it once and pay no more attention to it. Kindness to self and other both require coming back to, time and again.

In the previous chapter, we have portrayed how being compassionate means recognising and acknowledging suffering, expressing empathy, respect, and warmth, honouring patients' needs and wishes, and supporting them and their families. We have also underscored the beneficial influence it has on both patient and doctor.

Compassion exercises have been part of Buddhist traditional practice for more than 2,500 years (Epstein, 2017). These exercises, practiced regularly, cultivate kindness, care, and compassion as a way of being.

Can practicing compassion train people to be kind and caring?

Research has demonstrated that compassion practice influences parts of the brain that are correlated with understanding and resonating with others feelings, regulating our emotions, and expanding emotional compass (Engen & Singer, 2015; Weng, 2013).

The following exercises are derived from traditional Buddhist tradition, and are intended to expand our natural compassion as human beings in general, and doctors in particular. The exercises are based on the basic premise that we are all connected to each other, and each of us is a human being who copes with suffering and pain; has hopes and dreams; is trying to be happy. In these exercises, after relaxing, we bring to mind an image or a felt sense of someone and emanating feelings of gratitude and kindness. We try to look at the image of the other like a mother seeing her baby. We start with an exercise towards a benefactor, who is someone that embodies and inspires the quality of kindness in us. We go on with a neutral patient, someone with whom we struggle to emotionally engage, a patient for whom we have neither a strong positive feeling, nor negative ones. We end the exercise with compassion towards the difficult patient, someone who evokes in us intricate feelings and tests the limits of our empathy and compassion (Morgan & Morgan, 2005).

Exercise: Cultivating Compassion

Sit comfortably, allowing your eyes to gently close if it feels right.

Take a few moments to feel your body as a whole, and the sensations associated with touch in the places you are in contact with the floor. Let your attention settle on your breath, feel the rising and falling of your chest and abdomen.

Remind yourself that all human beings are interconnected, and each one of us copes with suffering and pain, has hopes and dreams, and trying to be happy.

Bring to mind a visual image or a felt sense of a benefactor. Imagine that he is sitting next to you. Look at him as a mother that looks at her newborn.

Direct at him feelings of gratitude and kindness.

When your mind wanders, gently return to this image and start again.

Be mindful and curious regarding your own sensations, feelings, and thoughts.

Do the same exercise with a neutral patient and afterwards with a difficult one.

If you find it difficult to generate these feelings, imagine that your benefactor is sitting next to you and send warmth to both of them.

Be curious and mindful about your interactions with difficult patients. Let them be your teachers that carry helpful insights for you.

In addition to these exercises that bestow us with compassionate approach when practiced regularly, the next exercise is useful when a patient comes in, and you want to reconnect with your empathy and compassion.

Exercise: Reconnecting with Your Compassion[1]

Take a few moments to feel your body as a whole, and the sensations associated with touch in the places you are in contact with the floor. Let your attention settle on your breath, feel the rising and falling of your chest and abdomen.

Concentrate on your intention to open your heart fully, be present, empathic, and compassionate.

Bring to your mind the understanding that all human beings are interconnected, and each one of us copes with suffering and pain, has hopes and dreams, and tries to be happy.

> *When you walk to the door, remind yourself that on the other side of the door, another human being is waiting for you with hope that you can relieve in some way his suffering.*
> *Remind yourself of the healing potential of human presence, empathy, and compassion.*
> *Open the door and greet your patient.*

In summary, human presence, empathy, and compassion are interconnected qualities that nurture, and when in balance have favourable benefits affecting both doctors and patients. Cultivating these precious qualities requires intention and practice, which will establish the conditions that avow empathy, compassion, and kindness to evolve.

Note

1. Based on the Metta Bhavana Buddhist meditation.

References

Charon, R. (2001). Narrative medicine: A model for empathy, reflection, profession and trust. *Journal of American Medical Association, 286*, 1897–902.

Coles, R. (1989). *The call of stories* (pp. 117–118). Boston, MA: Houghton Mifflin.

DasGupta, S., & Charon, R. (2004). Personal illness narratives: Using reflective writing to teach empathy. *Academic Medicine, 79*(4), 351–356.

Engen, H.G., & Singer, T. (2015). Compassion-based emotion regulation up-regulates experienced positive affect and associated neural networks. *Social Cognitive and Affective Neuroscience, 10*(9), 1291–1301.

Epstein, R.M. (2017). *Attending: Medicine, mindfulness and humanity*. New York, NY: Scribner.

Halpern, J. (2001). *From detached concern to empathy: Humanizing medical practice*. New York, NY: Oxford University Press.

Morgan, W.D., & Morgan, S.T. (2005). Cultivating attention and empathy. In C.K. Germer, R.D. Siegel, & P.R. Fulton (Eds.), *Mindfulness and psychotherapy* (pp. 73–90). New York, NY: Guilford Press.

Platt, F.W., & Keller V.F. (1994). Empathic communication: A teachable and learnable skill. *Journal of General Internal Medicine, 9*(4), 222–226.

Reiss, H. (2010). Empathy in medicine: A neurobiological perspective. *Journal of American Medical Association, 304*(14), 1604–1605.

Stern, D.N. (2004). *The present moment in psychotherapy and everyday life*. New York, NY: W.W. Norton & Co.

Taigman, M. (1996). Can empathy and compassion be taught? *Journal of Emergency Medical Services, 21*(6), 42–43, 25–46, 48.

Weng, H.Y. (2013). Compassion training altruism and neural responses to suffering. *Psychological Science, 24*(7), 1171–1180.

Part III

With the Body in Mind

Incorporating Body-Mind Skills in
Medical Treatment

12 The Body-Mind Connection

From Maimonides to Psychoneuroimmunoendocrinology

Barbara was a seventy-two-year-old woman, who was admitted to the hospital with chest pain and non-specific ECG changes. I first met her as a young medical student, more than twenty years ago. She was my first patient. I sat beside her and took a thorough medical history; conducted meticulous physical examinations; looked over her blood tests, chest X-ray, and her ECG. While taking her medical history, I noticed that she was simultaneously diagnosed with diabetes mellitus, hypertension, and psoriasis about ten years before. Curiously, I asked her about any special events in her life that had happened before. "Of course,", she said, "I retired after working for twenty-five years as a midwife, and my husband died a few months previously".

Those days, there was no reference to the body-mind connection in medical school, and its implications on clinical practice. Introducing my patient to the professor, I mentioned those stressful life events that preceded her medical diagnoses. I was embarrassed and ashamed, when the professor looked at me with wrathful eyes, and asked me if it had any relevance to the clinical decisions we have to make now, and accused me for wasting our time.

While the interaction of psychic and somatic processes has been questioned and studied for years, it was actually not long ago that medical sciences separated the mind from the body sustaining a dualistic approach. Based on scientific developments in recent years, the interaction of emotions and illness is now well recognised in the medical field.

This chapter will present an updated review of scientific and clinical research in psychoneuroimmunoendocrinology, neuroscience, and the impact of stress, depression, and trauma on health. Additionally, we will introduce you to the field of body psychotherapy, which endows us with a large body of knowledge and understanding of mind-body function. We believe that interweaving the two disciplines, medicine and psychotherapy, has the potential to shed more light on the complexity of this issue, and expand our understanding and options of application in clinical practice. Furthermore, we argue that body-psychotherapy, with its particular emphasis on mind-body connections and its myriad of physical, as well as psychological skills, is an especially relevant bridge between the two fields—medicine and psychotherapy.

12.1 The History of the Body-Mind Connection

The complex connection between psyche and soma has been a central interest and concern for centuries.

Prior to the evolution of the western medicine's dualistic view, body and mind unity was perceived as an undifferentiated whole. In those days, individuals sought relief for their mental, emotional, and spiritual maladies through healers, pastors, and shamans in their communities, who attributed illness and suffering to disconnection of the soul or the psyche from the body (Pickren, 2014).

Traditional therapies such as Chinese medicine, Yoga, and Tai Chi are based on the apprehension that the person represents a body-mind whole which cannot be reduced to somatic language or a psychological one. For instance, according to traditional Chinese medicine, emotional and bodily expressions are not detached or differentiated from each other (Connelly, 1994; Rolef Ben-Shahar, 2014). The twelfth-century doctor, philosopher, and Jewish leader Maimonides, who was one of the most famous medical doctors in history, discussed in his book *Regimen of Health* the connection between mental and physical health, particularly in relation to stress and anxiety. His ideas referring to the body and mind constitute the foundation of the psychosomatic medicine (Mizrahi, 2011).

In the seventeenth century, Descartes' influential philosophy, which is seen as the dawn of modern Western thinking, identified the self with its cognitive and thinking functioning—what is often known as the cogito (*cogito ergo sum*, I think therefore I am) (Descartes, 1636). This identification, which freed science to investigate the body without remaining accountable to the limiting hands of the church, also gave rise to a dualistic conception splitting between body and mind. The body became a corporeal machine and a platform for objective science, while the psyche was attributed to spiritual dimensions, and thus the domain of the church. The advent of Western medicine and empirical science have yielded inspiring achievements in medical care, while at the same time psychologic sciences have rendered remarkable contributions regarding the psyche. While these seminal accomplishments have major impact on physical and mental health, they also enhance body-mind dualism and separate us from our embodied experience (Capra, 1975).

Advances in the fields of psychosomatic medicine and psychoneuroimmunoendocrinology as well as in cognitive science and psychological studies have brought changing perspectives to the study of body-mind connection, and broadened our understanding and clinical implications thereof. Psychosomatic medicine is today an interdisciplinary field that deals with the interaction between biological, psychological, and social factors influencing the onset of diseases and their course. While psychosomatic medicine approach is primarily applied through verbal discursive relationship, the field of body psychotherapy comprises particular body-mind techniques and cultivates a unique attunement and ways of directly listening to bodily symptoms (Michalsen et al., 2012; Young, 2011).

We believe that integrating these two evolving disciplines could enrich our understanding of body-mind interaction, pave the scientific ground for the translation into clinical practice, and expand clinical implications significantly.

12.2 Psychosomatic Medicine: Clinical and Scientific Review

Psychosomatic medicine is a clinical and scientific field, founded on the concept that mind and body are integral aspects of human function. The main goals of the psychosomatic approach include building bridges between psych and soma, overcoming the mind-body dichotomy, understanding the interactions among biologic, psychologic, and social aspects in every patient, and developing a system based perspective and knowledge based on clinical and scientific research (Fritzsche, 2014).

Psychoneuroimmunoendocrinology

Psychoneuroimmunoendocrinology is an evolving multidisciplinary field, encompassing and elucidating the interactions among behaviours and the nervous, immune, and endocrine systems. Studies provide scientific evidence to these complex networks that communicate with each other, monitor and regulate a myriad of physiological functions, and contribute to the understanding of disease vulnerability (Nemeroff, 2013; Yan, 2016).

Recent studies explicate the complex processes involving the endocrine and neurotransmitter systems associated with the immune system, catecholamines, glucocorticoids, endorphins, and other neuropeptides, triggered by stress, depression, and negative emotions. While acute stress responses hold a protective and adaptive function, chronic stress may impair adaptive processes, affect the immune system, elevate proinflammatory cytokines, influence the hypothalamic-pituitary-adrenal (HPA) axis as well as sympathetic-adrenal-medullary axes (Goncharova & Tarakanov, 2007; Leonard & Myint, 2009).

Early life trauma, child abuse, and neglect all increase risk for depression, anxiety disorders, and a variety of medical conditions. Such traumatic history acts upon the developing the central nervous system, producing structural changes in the brain and in neurotransmitter systems, which correlate with a variety of psychiatric symptoms and higher risk of diseases (Cisler et al., 2013; Gould et al., 2012; Heim et al., 2010, 2013). Individual differences in stress reactivity, patterns of personalities, coping styles, as well as emotional and cognitive responses are associated with a host of physiological responses and homeostasis, including a variety of immunity-related states, and therefore have significant role in medical conditions (Cacioppo & Berntson, 2007; Kemeny, 2007).

The "Second Brain"

In addition to the brain, the enteric nervous system, which is the intrinsic nervous system of the gut, made up of an extensive network of neurons and neurotransmitters, is also referred to as the "second brain" of the body (Gershon, 1999). Recent neurobiological discoveries regarding this gut-brain crosstalk have revealed a complex, bidirectional communication system that as well as assuring the maintenance of gastrointestinal homeostasis and digestion, is also responsible for multiple effects on affect, motivation, and higher cognitive functions. Innervations of sympathetic and parasympathetic nerves regulate intestinal function and mediate emotion-related patterns of regional changes in motor, secretory, and possibly immune activity in the gastrointestinal tract (Mayer, 2011). When facing threat and stress, this complex gut-brain system is triggered and shifts to sympathetic nervous system response (Music, 2015; Davis, 2018).

Epigenetics

Body-mind connections are also found in regulation of gene activities. Epigenetic mechanisms transduce environmental inputs, like stress, into physiological and behavioural change. Stress has a number of known effects on epigenetic marks in the brain, generating shifts in processes such as DNA methylation and histone modifications (Hunter, 2012; Hunter & McEwen, 2013; Hunter et al., 2015). In other words, the DNA sequence remains the same, but the genes' activity changes remarkably, and therefore the functionality of the brain and other organs are affected, and have the potential to trigger psychosomatic disorders (Fritzsche, 2014).

Clinical Research

On the clinical level, stress and depression have been related to cardiovascular diseases, obesity, diabetes, various types of cancer, neurodegenerative diseases, rheumatoid arthritis, and a variety of skin diseases (Ho et al., 2010; Leonard & Myint, 2009; Nemeroff, 2013; Shelton & Miller, 2010; Tausk et al., 2008). Psychosomatic clinical research shows a number of factors modulating individual vulnerability. Stressful life events in the year preceding the onset of symptoms of a number of medical conditions, has been observed (Fink, 2016; Novack et al., 2007). Other important factors are health attitudes and behaviour, social support, and psychological well-being (Fava et al., 2017).

While these mechanisms underscore the magnitude of stress, depression, and personality traits in vulnerability of a myriad of health conditions and their course, research has not proved to be the conceptual panacea initially hoped for by some psychologists and immunologists (Ouellette & DiPlacido, 2001). Some of the well-controlled studies of personality, stress, and illness fail to find comprehensive psycho-immunological mediating mechanisms (Kemeny,

2007). Moreover, while antidepressant medications used for treating depression in the setting of medical disease was found effective in reducing psychiatric symptoms, their effect on improving medical outcomes was not demonstrated (Jackson et al., 2004; Rackley & Bostwick, 2012). Friedman (2007) proposes that this complexity might originate from multiple causal links including stress and behavioural and biological connections operating concurrently, and with different stages across time. He explains that current research in psychoneuroimmunoendocrinology expounds only one important mediating mechanism between the individual and the health outcome. He asserts that integration into the broader conceptual understandings of personality and health, using a new lifespan epidemiological personality approach is essential.

We opine that a discrete explanatory theory derived from a psychological model, dealing with the interface of emotion and somatic functions, could provide a broader framework for research and practical implications in medical practice.

In the next section we will introduce the modality of body psychotherapy and elaborate on the concepts and practical applications regarding body-mind connection.

12.3 Body Psychotherapy

Body psychotherapy is a distinct branch of psychotherapy with a long history and a large body of literature and knowledge based upon a sound theoretical position. Originated with a few students-turned-colleagues of Freud who felt that psychological issues were both manifesting in, and were deeply entwined with, physiological processes and that separating the two was an ill-advised and inefficient practice (Ferenczi, 1929; Groddeck, 1931; Reich, 1933). It includes a variety of theoretical and clinical methodologies, as well as different styles of therapeutic interventions and toolkits based on a theory of mind-body functioning, which takes into account the complexity of the intersections and interactions between the body and the mind. The common underlying assumption is that the body is the whole person, and there is a functional unity (in Reich's 1933, terminology) between mind and body. Body psychotherapy views the relationship between corporal and psychological processes as both unified and complementary, that is—it is not a hierarchical relationship, but two manifestations of the same organism. Body (somatic processes) and mind (cognitive emotional processes) are both seen as functioning and interactive aspects of the whole human being, while the body is involved in the process of making meaning. Body psychotherapists use somatic attunement skills to deepen their awareness of themselves and their patients' bodies; they cultivate the process of bridge building, and connecting body and mind, feelings, sensations, and thoughts; they perceive bodily symptoms as carrying emotional and cognitive meaning, and use a number of bodily interventions (breathing techniques, mindfulness, grounding, and centring) for coping with stress, pain, and other symptoms (Bucci, 1997; Lin & Payne, 2014; Rolef Ben-Shahar, 2014; Young, 2011).

To reiterate, when a patient comes in with a bodily symptom, whether medically explained or not, I perceive the symptom as a part of a larger context, which includes cognitive, emotional, and somatic dimensions, as well as societal and cultural. Therefore, I am attuned to both verbal and nonverbal expressions of the experience. Through the body psychotherapy lens (but also systemic and analytic perspectives), the symptom functions as a nonverbal channel expressing a deeper and wider process (Bucci, 1997; Keeney, 1983; Morgan, 1996; Westland, 2015). I might use body-mind interventions that might deepen connection between the symptom and other dimensions of the experience, a process which might broaden the understanding and meaning, and use other techniques useful for alleviating pain and stress.

12.4 Building Bridges: Integrative Medicine

Psychosomatic interventions include cultivation of the doctor-patient relationship, assessment of psychosocial factors which might affect illness vulnerability, prevention strategies, health behaviour modifications, psychotherapeutic interventions, and pharmacotherapy (Fava et al., 2017). Expressing it succinctly, we may say that integrative medicine is medicine within its broader context. While these significant validated interventions are based on primarily verbal discursive relationship, mind-body medicine applies various nonverbal interventions based on traditional practices such as relaxation, yoga, and mindfulness. The combination of the two disciplines in a clinical context, addressed as integrative medicine, holds the potential of being complementary and synergistic (Michalsen et al., 2012). However, this approach is far from being translated into operational steps in clinical practice for many reasons—among them are lack of time, inappropriate training, and insufficient existing applicable interventions to be use in the clinical setting.

Based on our own clinical experience, we will try, in the following chapters to integrate substantial knowledge derived from body psychotherapy into the existing models, in a way that we believe can elaborate and enrich the integrative medical approach, and enclose practical elementary interventions in the medical encounter.

References

Bucci, W. (1997). Symptoms and symbols: A multiple code theory of somatization. *Psychoanalytic Inquiry, 17*, 151–172.

Cacioppo, J.T., & Berntson, G.G. (2007). The brain, homeostasis, and health: Balancing demands of the internal and external milieu. In H.S. Friedman & R.C. Silver (Eds.), *Foundations of health psychology* (pp. 73–91). New York, NY: Oxford University Press.

Capra, F. (1975). *The Tao of physics*. Boulder, CO: Shambala.

Cisler, J.M., James, G.A., Tripathi, S., Mletzko, T., Heim, C., Hu, X.P., . . . Kilts, C.D. (2013). Differential functional connectivity within an emotion regulation neural network among individuals resilient and susceptible to the depressogenic effects of early life stress. *Psychological Medicine, 43*(3), 507–518.

Connelly, D.M. (1994). *Traditional acupuncture: The law of the five elements* (2nd ed.). Columbia, SC: Traditional Acupuncture Institute.

Davis, E.A. (2018). Investigation of non-traditional roles of the neural gut-brain axis. PhD dissertation, University of Illinois at Urbana-Champaign.

Descartes, R. (1636). Discourse on method. In M.D. Wilson (Ed.), *The essential Descartes*. New York, NY: Meridian, 1983.

Fava, G.A., Cosci, F., & Sonino, N. (2017). Current psychosomatic practice. *Psychotherapy and Psychosomatics, 86*(1), 13–30.

Ferenczi, S. (1929). The principle of relaxation and neocatharsis. In S. Ferenczi & M. Balint (Eds.), *Final contributions to the problems and methods of psychoanalysis*. London: Maresfield Reprints, 1980.

Fink, G. (2016). Stress neuroendocrinology: Highlights and controversies. In *Stress: Neuroendocrinology and neurobiology* (pp. 1–15). New York, NY: Academic Press.

Friedman, H.S. (2007). The multiple linkages of personality and disease. *Brain, Behavior, and Immunity, 22*(5), 668–675.

Fritzsche, K. (2014). What is psychosomatic medicine? In K. Fritzsche, S.H. McDaniel, & M. Wirsching (Eds.), *Psychosomatic medicine: An international primer for primary care setting* (pp. 3–12). New York, NY: Springer Publishing Company.

Gershon, M. (1999). The enteric system: A second brain. *Hospital Practice, 34*(31-32).

Goncharova, L.B., & Tarakanov, A.O. (2007). Molecular networks of brain and immunity. *Brain Research Reviews, 55*(1), 155–166.

Gould, F., Clarke, J., Heim, C., Harvey, P.D., Majer, M., & Nemeroff, C.B. (2012). The effects of child abuse and neglect on cognitive functioning in adulthood. *Journal of Psychiatric Research, 46*, 500–506.

Groddeck, G. (1931). Psychic conditioning and the psychoanalytic treatment of organic disorders. In L. Schnacht (Ed.), *The meaning of illness: Selected psychoanalytic writings* by Georg Groddeck. London: Maresfield Library, 1977.

Heim, C.M., Mayberg, H.S., Mletzko, T., Nemeroff, C.B., & Pruessner, J.C. (2013). Decreased cortical representation of genital somatosensory field after childhood sexual abuse. *American Journal of Psychiatry, 170*(6), 616–623.

Heim, C.M., Shugart, M., Craighead, W.E., & Nemeroff, C.B. (2010). Neurobiological and psychiatric consequences of child abuse and neglect. *Developmental Psychobiology, 52*, 671–690.

Ho, R.C.M., Neo, L.F., Chua, A.N.C., Check, A.A., & Mak, A. (2010). Research on psychoneuroimmunology: Does stress influence immunity and cause coronary artery disease? *Annals of the Academy of Medicine, Singapore, 39*, 191–196.

Hunter, R.G. (2012). Epigenetic effects of stress and corticosteroids in the brain. *Frontiers in Cellular Neuroscience, 6*, 18.

Hunter, R.G., Gagnidze, K., McEwen, B.S., & Pfaff, D.W. (2015). Stress and the dynamic genome: Steroids, epigenetics, and the transposome. *Proceedings of the National Academy of Sciences, 112*(22), 6828–6833.

Hunter, R.G., & McEwen, B.S. (2013). Stress and anxiety across the lifespan: Structural plasticity and epigenetic regulation. *Epigenomics, 5*, 177–194.

Jackson, J.L., de Zee, K., & Berbano, E. (2004). Can treating depression improve disease outcomes? *Annals of Internal Medicine, 140*, 1054–1056.

Keeney, B. (1983). *Aesthetics of change*. New York, NY: Guilford Press.

Kemeny, M.E. (2007). Psychoneuroimmunology. In H.S. Friedman & R.C. Silver (Eds.), *Foundations of health psychology* (pp. 92–116). New York, NY: Oxford University Press.

Leonard, B.E., & Myint, A. (2009). The psychoneuroimmunology of depression. *Human Psychopharmacology, 24*, 165–175.

Lin, Y., & Payne, H. (2014). The BodyMind Approach™, medically unexplained symptoms and personal construct psychology. *Body, Movement and Dance in Psychotherapy, 9*(3), 154–166.

Mayer, E.A. (2011). Gut feelings: The emerging biology of gut-brain communication. *Nature Reviews Neuroscience, 12*, 453–466.

Michalsen, A., Traitteur, H., Lüdtke, R., Brunnhuber, S., Meier, L., Jeitler, M., Büssing, A., & Kessler, C. (2012). Yoga for chronic neck pain: a pilot randomized controlled clinical trial. *The Journal of Pain, 13*(11), 1122–1130.

Mizrahi, A. (2011). The soul and the body in the philosophy of the Rambam. *Rambam Maimonides Medical Journal, 2*(2).

Morgan, D. (1996). *The principles of hypnotherapy*. Bradford, England: Eildon Press.

Music, G. (2015). Bringing up the bodies: Psych-soma, body awareness and feeling at ease. *British Journal of Psychotherapy, 31*(1), 4–19.

Nemeroff, C.B. (2013). Psychoneuroimmunoendocrinology: The biological basis of mind-body physiology and pathophysiology. *Depression and Anxiety, 30*, 285–287.

Novack, D.H., Cameron, O., Epel, E., Ader, R., Waldstein, S.R., Levenstein, S., . . . Wainer, A.R. (2007). Psychosomatic medicine: The scientific foundation of the biopsychosocial model. *Academic Psychiatry, 31*, 388–401.

Ouellette, S.C., & DiPlacido, J. (2001). Personality's role in the protection and enhancement of health: Where the research has been, where it is stuck, how it might move. In A. Baum, T.A. Revenson, & J. Singer (Eds.), *Handbook of health psychology* (pp. 175–194). Hillsdale, NJ: Lawrence Erlbaum Associates.

Pickren, W. (2014). *The psychology book: From Shamanism to cutting edge neuroscience, 250 milestones in the history of psychology*. New York, NY: Sterling Publishing.

Rackley, S., & Bostwick, J.M. (2012). Depression in medically ill patients. *Psychiatric Clinics of North America, 35*(1), 231–247.

Reich, W. (1933). *Character analysis*. New York, NY: Noonday Press, 1972.

Rolef Ben-Shahar, A. (2014). *Touching the relational edge: Body psychotherapy*. London: Karnac Books.

Shelton, R.C., & Miller, A.H. (2010). Eating ourselves to death (and despair): The contribution of adiposity and inflammation to depression. *Progress in Neurobiology, 91*, 275–299.

Tausk, F., Elenkov, I., & Moynihan, J. (2008). Psychoneuroimmunology. *Dermatology and Therapy, 21*, 22–31.

Westland, G. (2015). *Verbal and non-verbal communication in psychotherapy*. New York, NY: W.W. Norton & Co.

Yan, Q. (2016). *Stress and inflammation: A systems biology perspective*: Psychoneuroimmunology: *Systems biology approaches to mind-body medicine*. New York, NY: Springer Publishing Company.

Young, C. (2011). The science of body psychotherapy today: Part 1: A background history. In C. Young (Ed.), *About the science of body psychotherapy* (pp. 25–50). Stow, Scotland: Body Psychotherapy Publications.

13 The Language of the Body

The Psych Speaks the Soma

He has been coughing for more than a year. Days and nights, the cough won't stop. Chest X-ray, chest CT, allergy tests, and blood tests are all normal except from a mild obstruction in pulmonary functions. He has tried different kinds of inhalers, corticosteroids, and antihistamines to no avail. It is the third time I meet Julian. He is a fifty-year-old hairdresser, who has just moved in town. He keeps telling me how exhausted he is, and pleads for my help. I read again his medical history and ask him further questions regarding his symptoms and his life. He answers my questions quietly and politely, avoiding eye contact. There is nothing new, the same old details, and no new data about his life. I feel anxious and helpless. How can I help him?

I take a pause, finding a moment to breathe, to help me feel and think more clearly. I look back at Julian, his bowed head supported by his hands and his crouched body fill me with a sense of despair. I seek for his eyes, when he glimpses, and for a brief moment our eyes meet. Looking at his black big agonizing eyes, I am imbued with sadness and sorrow.

"You look sad, Julian", I tell him.

He turns his gaze away from me, looking down. We are both silent for a moment.

"I am", he suddenly whispers.

"Would you like to tell me more?" I ask.

"No use", he murmurs, "he's gone".

"What happened, Julian?"

He is silent, his body shivering, and his head down.

"It's my son . . . you see, I have a son . . . I had a son . . ." he stammers, "He died a year ago."

His body contracts, he can hardly breathe.

"I am so sorry, Julian", I say softly feeling his agony.

He lifts his head up; his eyes are filled with anguish conflated with anger. "I will never forgive myself", he outcries grasping his wrists, " you see, he had tuberculosis, he couldn't stop coughing day and night . . . nothing helped . . . and I . . . I just couldn't. . . . I couldn't bear the sound of his cough anymore . . .".

He is shaking, tears in his eyes, "and now . . ." he cries," I'll do anything to hear his cough once again . . ."

While patients' experience of symptoms does not follow the body-mind split that features the classification of disease in medical practice, doctors get to know them through their education based on model experiences linked to determined diseases (Davidsen et al., 2016; Rudebeck, 2000). Acquiring knowledge and skills in medical training is mediated through anatomy, laboratories, and functions of the body which are outlined comprehensively. Nevertheless, patients often display diffuse and vague symptoms that do not match bodily or mental categories. In life, the contextual and multifaceted nature of our being is far more intertwined than any single discipline could describe.

There are several theoretical approaches to understanding patients with symptoms which do not fit into somatic or psychic category. Engel's biopsychosocial model which comprises psychological and social aspects in the understanding of the patient (Engel, 1977, 1980) has been subject for criticism for holding a dualistic view of human experience (Borrell-Carrio et al., 2004; Ghaemi, 2009). Rudebeck (2000) asserts that when doctors encounter their patients' symptoms, they set out their "biomedical reflex" (p. 4), and they tend to look for facts that support their initial diagnostic hypothesis. He also argues that whereas the psychosomatic attitude might be a useful diagnostic tool and a research perspective with a holistic intent, it does not familiarise the doctor with the patient's unique experience. He explains that the psychosomatic approach underscores diseases rather than experiences, and accentuates observation rather than interaction. Simply put, to fully understand the broad human context of our patients, we are called to bring the most complex and nonlinear diagnostic tool we have, our own humanity. Alongside every piece of data and skill we have, it is through ourselves as human organisms who are willing to interact with the other as a human organism that we can learn about their pains, hopes, and potential paths to recovery and healing.

In a study conducted by Davidsen (2009), she illustrates how primary care physicians differ in their approach to symptoms presentations. Her research depicts two kinds of doctors: (1) therapeutically minded doctors who follow the patient's experience and carry out bodily examinations, yet are simultaneously open to the possibility that symptoms do not originate from a bodily pathology and might refer the patient to psychiatric consultation; (2) dismissive doctors who dismiss the option of bodily pathology by saying that the problem derives from the mind. She elucidates that both kinds of doctors express a mind-body dualism by operating with a division between the physical and the psychic and separating consultations with the patients about physical or psychological problems.

Some theoretical models have attempted to overcome this complexity. According to Balint's integrative view, patient's symptoms can lead to different understandings of the illnesses, depending on the way the patient as a whole is encountered by the doctor, and on the interaction between them (Balint, 1964). McWhinney (1996) has formulated an integrative approach based on Balint's view of the person as a whole, and the realisation that understanding patients' symptoms can be established in an intersubjective interaction that does not distinguish between physical and mental dimensions as completely separate.

Davidsen and his colleagues (2016) signify the complexity of understanding patients' undifferentiated symptoms and stresses the significance of understanding their experience and sensations instead of jumping to diagnostic conclusions or categorising into mental or physical phenomena. Rudebeck (2000) perceives symptom presentations as unique act of communicating existential messages that hold meanings. He thinks that in order to approach patients' experience, doctors need a language that can give meaning to diseases without using medical terms.

Julian's cough is a good example of a symptom presentation that communicates his emotional deep pain, with both physiologic dimension (mild pulmonary obstruction) and psychological one. The possibility to engage with Julian's whole experience expressed by his body, his affect, and the content of our conversation, enabled the meaning of his cough to unfold and opened a broader understanding of his refractory cough. It took about two months for the cough to be replaced gradually by a painful process of grief. But even if we are reluctant to consider Julian's symptoms as psychosomatically created, we can surely agree that the meaning attributed to the symptoms strongly affects the patient's cooperation, the implementation of the physician's prescription, and therefore the prospect of recovery. Healing, like illness, is context-sensitive, and we wish to suggest that sensitivity to that context can make us better doctors, whether we hold a holistic worldview or not.

Body psychotherapy views bodily symptoms and pain as neither somatic nor psychic, but carrying both aspects. It understands people as psychosomatic systems, and therefore every physical symptom has a psychological expression and every emotional happening manifests physically. In other words, any symptom, pain, or disease is psychosomatic, and the relationship between these two dimensions is not causal or hierarchical, but complementary and dialectic—our thinking and feeling manifest in our somatic reality, and vice versa—our bodily changes affect and interact with our cognitive and emotional realities (Rolef Ben-Shahar, 2014). Body psychotherapy proposes an interaction between body and emotions, where symptoms constitute a language with encoded messages that might provide a bridge to deeper knowledge (Kashi-kark, 2011).

We believe that interweaving body psychotherapy's point of view together with particular skills of listening to the body's language could broaden and enrich medical practice. In the next sections we will present the difference between verbal and body languages, explain how the body speaks the psyche, and introduce a broadened attitude towards medically unexplained symptoms and chronic pain.

13.1 The Organisation of the Human Experience

From cellular protein expressions to complex social behaviours, each human experience is organised and articulated by somatic, emotional, cognitive, and relational aspects, with each facet influencing the other. That is to say that the body may reveal mental-emotional issues and mental-emotional activity might be recorded throughout the body (Rolef Ben-Shahar, 2014; Siegel, 2006).

In chapter 12 we discussed how mental attitudes, stress, and various emotions could constitute a full body event which affects the nervous system, immunologic functions, and endocrine activity (suffice is to think of how physically vulnerable we become following the death of a loved one). Together with cellular effects, these kinds of events affect sensations, feelings, breathing, muscles, posture, gestures, and more. In contrast to cellular effects that can be seldom assessed in laboratories or special imaging tests, these bodily manifestations can be sensed and perceived during an interactive encounter with our patients, and therefore serve as an aperture to the whole experience.

Let's return to Julian and examine the various dimensions of his experience. On the somatic level we can notice his hesitant eye contact, shiver, changes in his voice and breath, and changes in his muscles affecting his posture and gestures (e.g., head down, grasping feasts). On the emotional level we can feel his helplessness, sadness, agony, and guilt, and on the cognitive level we can realise how far he is from forgiving himself. Societal and cultural perspectives could also be thought of here, in terms of functioning, nuclear family and broader social network and more. Looking at Julian's cough as a symptom that does not have to be categorised as either somatic or psychological, but as an expression of a broader experience, makes it possible to find more adjusted interventions which might assist him better. He welcomes the process of meaning giving to his symptoms, which has not only allowed him to recover physically, but has also supported him in his grief over the death of his son. In order to approach his experience, it was not enough to hear the content of the conversation and taking biopsychosocial anamnesis, but it was required to listen to non-verbal language that led to the understanding of the full experience.

13.2 Verbal Language Versus Non-Verbal Language

In order to converge with the patient's experience, we need to be familiar with verbal and nonverbal languages and be attuned to both. As social creatures, we do so naturally. We tend to believe someone's body language more than their words when the two contradict one another. Information is represented in mind in a verbal mode and a nonverbal one as well (Bucci, 1997). The verbal mode is mediated via the language of words and meanings. Patients express their symptoms, thoughts, emotions, and subjective experience through verbal languages. Nowadays, more than ever, patients also communicate the meaning they attribute to their symptoms. As doctors, we are used to listen to this form of communication; we ask a myriad of open and close questions in an attempt to understand our patients, make the right diagnosis, and tailor the best treatment for them.

In parallel to the verbal system, there are multiple channels of a nonverbal system. As doctors, we are experts in observing bodily manifestations such as colour of skin, heart rate, blood pressure, swellings, rashes, etc., all are indicators of the presence of a medical condition or its absence. Most experienced doctors, for example, are excellent lie detectors. Nonetheless, nonverbal language is also uttered as body movements, facial expressions, and gestures, breathing patterns, sensations, and symptoms (Bucci, 2008; Fogel, 2009; Gendlin, 1962). To successfully communicate with the somatic language, we need to listen to the body's own language, and value the input we receive from this type of communication. Somatic cues accompany the patient's words and reveal meanings which augment, elaborate, or contradict what the patient communicates verbally (Arlow, 1979; Bucci, 2001).

Listening to these somatic manifestations as a language that expresses meanings would shed light on a variety of aspects. First, it would facilitate a better understanding of how the patient perceives and addresses his symptoms (Is he anxious? Is he indifferent?). The way patients feel about their symptoms and diagnoses have tremendous impact on their well-being, cooperation, and, therefore, on the course of their diseases. Since patients often conceal their fears, helplessness, and other emotions in the medical encounter, perusing nonverbal indicators for their emotional experience is of paramount experience. Second, bodily language can provide us with information regarding to the quality of the relationship we have created with our patients, which has already shown in previous chapters, is of utmost importance. Third (and the core of our discussion in this chapter), listening to the body language enables us to perceive a symptom as an expression of a wider and profound experience which is verbally unspoken and often unconscious; a way in which the soma speaks the psyche. By watching television for an hour on mute, and attempting to note what we learn about the speakers, we can begin to appreciate how expert we are in attending to nonverbal communication. Doing it consciously, and gaining knowledge and experience in this type of language can significantly improve our practice (and our communication in life too).

13.3 The Soma Speaks the Psyche

As already discussed, the interaction between mind and body is an ongoing multilayered process. While the body takes an active part in psychic processes manifested in cellular, physiological, epigenetic, and structural levels, it also has an active role in the process of making meanings (Koch et al., 2013). Rudebeck (2000) alleges that the body and its parts get their meanings based on their functions in life. He exemplifies how the walking legs hold meaning of independence, and sex organs symbolise masculinity or femininity. Therefore, he asserts that subjective symptom presentations render existential messages, which should be kept in mind within the diagnostic process.

Medically unexplained symptoms (MUS) refer to the bodily complaints of patients when aetiology is unclear but produces significant psychological distress. Symptoms often do not follow anatomic or physiologic patterns and tend to be diffuse (Fritzsche, 2014). Patients can be diagnosed as suffering from MUS when symptoms are consistent for at least 6 months and significantly disturb their quality of life (Payne & Stott, 2010). It was previously been described as 'Somatoform disorder', and has been renamed as Somatic Symptom Disorder in DSM-V (American Psychiatric Association, 2013).

MUS are very common current complaints in primary care, with about 20% of patients consulting their family physician with limited effective treatments (Burton, 2003; Fritzsche, 2014; Kirmayer et al., 2004; Kroenke, 2007). It is widely recognised that MUS are psychologically related, with several psychosocial factors known to promote somatisation such as childhood trauma, negative bonding experience, model learning from parental models experiencing similar complaints, anxiety, and depression (Brown, 2004; Fritzsche, 2014; Payne, 2009; Wayne & Edward, 1998).

Despite the fact that MUS constitute a complex combination of both physical and psychological dimensions, the concept of MUS fosters a dualistic approach in which patients' symptoms are perceived as either organic (i.e., medically explained) or psychological (i.e., medically unexplained—the infamous 'it's all in your head').

Doctors, who listen carefully to their patients' narratives and experience of symptoms, are acquainted with the feeling that a certain symptom holds a deeper meaning in the patient's life. A young man presenting with low back pain, who copes with a major conflict regarding his career; a young woman with a history of sexually abuse and frequent migraines, which showed up after the beginning of an intimate relationship with a man, are two common variations of this phenomena.

How can we understand this process?

Conversion is a central concept described in early psychoanalytic thinking that refers to a process in which intolerable dissociated psychic pain converts into a symptomatic bodily expression (Brown, 2004; Breuer & Freud, 1957). Traumatic experiences can create intense insufferable pain, which is too difficult to process psychologically, and consequently is dissociated and then converted to a symptom. In other words, bodily symptoms might be perceived as a defence mechanism in which psychological distress is expressed without conscious awareness. From this perspective, Julian's cough gives voice to his unspeakable and unprocessed pain and guilt regarding his son's demise.

This model has been expanded with a theoretical background established, enabling exploration of the body's role in the process of making meaning (Bucci, 1997; Lin & Payne, 2014; McDougall & Coen, 2000).

Bucci (1997), referring the verbal and nonverbal systems, comprehended these defences as forms of disconnection between these two systems. She suggested that a particular bodily part or process might function as a symbol of an emotional experience which has been dissociated in the service of defence. Similarly, McDougall and Coen (2000) pled that traumatic affects that could not be encoded in verbal language, might be registered within the body's memory, and then be expressed in bodily symptoms.

Lin and Payne (2014) illustrate how people might not be aware of their emotional pains and, therefore, are not capable of verbally speaking about them. They elaborate how these unspeakable issues could be referenced by bodily symptoms, which means that some of our traumatic experiences that are too painful for us to process, or imperil our existed psychological function would manifest as a body symptom later in life. Expanding the dissociation and conversion model, they propose that besides being dissociated and converted, traumatic events might be suspended and placed in low levels of awareness. That means that patients show a spectrum of awareness, with the higher the level is, so is the cognitive and emotional aspects more accessible.

In addition to painful experiences, people are not always aware of their desires, yearnings, and motivations, which when not verbally communicated might be articulated as bodily symptoms. In this way symptoms serve as a way to communicate unspoken wishes, desires, fears, and more. A common example is a child complaining of abdominal pain (which meets criteria of functional abdominal pain) every time he has to go to school. In many cases, the child does not lie, but actually experiences pain. Instead of communicating his difficulties at school verbally with his parents (or sometimes even being able to conceive them himself), his body takes the role.

Norma, a fifty-four-year-old patient of mine, suffering from an autoimmune disease, had recurrent flare-ups every time her husband had to go on a business trip. Each time he went away, her joints would become severely inflamed. While exploring together this "coincidence", she realised that instead of asking her husband to stay home, her body communicated her request nonverbally.

As we can see, listening to the body's language is crucial in medical practice; it has an important role in approaching the patient's whole experience; and it might reveal hidden and unconscious psychological issues and disclose relevant meanings that can affect significantly medical management.

In the next chapter we will introduce you with practical diagnostic tools that would help listen more efficiently and accurately to your patients' body language.

References

American Psychiatric Association. (2013). *Somatic symptom disorder*. Retrieved on 17 December 2013, from www.dsm5.org/Documents/Somatic%20Symptom%20 Disorder%

Arlow, J.A. (1979). The genesis of interpretation. *Journal of American Psychoanalytic Association, 27*, 193–206. Reprinted in Psychoanalysis: Clinical theory and practice (1991), Madison, CT: International Universities Press, pp. 279–288.

Balint, M. (1964). *The doctor, his patient and the illness* (2nd ed.). London: Pitman Medical Publishing.

Borrell-Carrio, F., Suchman, A.L., & Epstein, R.M. (2004). The biopsychosocial model 25 years later: Principles, practice, and scientific inquiry. *Annals of Family Medicine, 2*(6), 576–582.

Breuer, J., & Freud, S. (1957). *Studies on hysteria*. New York, NY: Basic Books.

Brown, R.J. (2004). Psychological mechanisms of medically unexplained symptoms: An integrative conceptual model. *Psychological Bulletin, 130*, 793–812.

Bucci, W. (2001). Pathways of emotional communication. *Psychoanalytic Inquiry, 21*, 40–70.

Bucci, W. (2008). The role of bodily experience in emotional organization. In F.S. Anderson (Ed.), *Bodies in treatment: The unspoken dimension* (pp. 51–76). Hove, East Sussex: Analytic Press.

Burton, C. (2003). Beyond somatisation: A review of the understanding and treatment of medically unexplained physical symptoms (MUPS). *British Journal of General Practice, 53*, 231–239.

Davidsen, A.S. (2009). How does the general practitioner understand the patient? A qualitative study about psychological interventions in general practice. *Psychology and Psychotherapy: Theory, Research and Practice, 82*(2), 199–217.

Davidsen, A.S., Guassora, A.D., & Reventlow, S. (2016). Understanding the body-mind in primary care. *Medicine, Health Care and Philosophy, 19*(4), 581–594.

Engel, G.L. (1977). The need for a new medical model: A challenge for biomedicine. *Science, 196*(4286), 129–136.

Engel, G.L. (1980). The clinical-application of the biopsychosocial model. *American Journal of Psychiatry, 137*(5), 535–544.

Fogel, A. (2009). *The psychophysiology of self-awareness*. New York, NY: W.W. Norton & Co.

Fritzsche, K. (2014). Somatoform disorders. In K. Fritzsche, S.H. McDaniel, & M. Wirsching (Eds.), *Psychosomatic medicine: An international primer for primary care setting* (pp. 111–129). New York, NY: Springer Publishing Company.

Gendlin, E.T. (1962). *Experiencing and the creation of meaning*. New York, NY: Free Press of Glencoe.

Ghaemi, S.N. (2009). The rise and fall of the biopsychosocial model. *British Journal of Psychiatry, 195*(1), 3–4.

Kashi-Kark, A. (2011). Knowing pain: *The effects of body psychotherapy treatment on a person dealing with chronic pain*. (Diploma in Body Psychotherapy thesis, Reidman College, Tel Aviv).

Kirmayer, L.J., Groleau, D., Looper, K.J., & Dominice´, M. (2004). Explaining medically unexplained symptoms. *The Canadian Journal of Psychiatry/La Revue Canadienne de Psychiatrie, 49*, 663–672.

Koch, A.C., Caldwell, C., & Fuchs, T. (2013). On body memory and embodied therapy. *Body, Movement and Dance in Psychotherapy, 8*, 82–94.

Kroenke, K. (2007). Efficacy of treatment for somatoform disorders: A review of randomized controlled trials. *Psychosomatic Medicine, 69*, 881–888.

Lin, Y., & Payne, H. (2014). The bodymind approach, medically unexplained symptoms and personal construct psychology. *Body, Movement and Dance in Psychotherapy, 9*(3), 154–166.

McDougall, J., & Coen, S.J. (2000). Affect, somatisation and symbolisation. *The International Journal of Psychoanalysis, 81*, 159–161.

McWhinney, I.R. (1996). The importance of being different. *British Journal of General Practice, 46*(408), 433–436.

McWhinney, I.R. (2000). Being a general practitioner: What it means. *European Journal of General Practice, 6*(4), 135–139.

Payne, H. (2009). The BodyMind Approach to psychotherapeutic groupwork with patients with medically unexplained symptoms: A review of the literature, description of approach and methodology selected for a pilot study. *European Journal for Counselling and Psychotherapy, 11*, 287–310.

Payne, H., & Stott, D. (2010). Change in the moving bodymind: Quantitative results from a pilot study on the BodyMind Approach (BMA) as groupwork for patients with medically unexplained symptoms (MUS). *Counselling and Psychotherapy Research, 10*, 295–307.

Rolef Ben-Shahar, A. (2014). *Touching the relational edge: Body psychotherapy.* London: Karnac Books.

Rudebeck, C.E. (2000). The doctor, the patient and the body. *Scandinavian Journal of Health Care, 18*, 4–8.

Siegel, D.J. (2006). An interpersonal neurobiology approach to psychotherapy: Awareness, mirror neurons, and well-being. *Psychiatric Annals, 36*, 248–256.

Wayne, J.K., & Edward, A.W. (1998). Medically unexplained symptoms in primary care. *Journal of Clinical Psychiatry, 59*, 15–21.

14 Listening to the Language of the Body

For more than a year, Rob has been complaining of diffuse annoying muscle pains. He is a forty-seven-year-old charismatic chief executive officer in a successful company. Physical examination, blood tests, EMG, and imaging tests were all normal. He has been oscillating from one specialist to another, trying different kinds of medications, undergoing various treatments offered in a pain clinic including acupuncture with no improvement.

Sitting in front of him, he stares at me with pleading eyes when he says, "You've got to help me. You are my family doctor after all. I thought about it. . . . Maybe it's a vitamin I need, I read about it in the internet".

My body draws back and shrinks. His beseeching gaze makes me feel ashamed and helpless. I have tried everything I know and referred him to the best specialists. When I inquire about his private life, he describes a happy marriage and satisfaction in his career. "It's just this irritating pain that drives me crazy", he keeps saying. "Everything else is OK, no unusual stress at home".

"So . . . what are you saying?" he asks, "Should I take vitamins? Perhaps another blood test?"

"Your blood tests results from last month are all normal, including your vitamins. There is no need to take more blood tests now", I say.

His begging eyes open widely, his breathing gets deeper and he straightens up. My breath tightens at his penetrating incensed look.

"So, what are you saying to me? Isn't there anything else to do?" he raises his voice. "Just don't tell me it is psychological, I am not depressed, I am a strong man, I haven't cried since the age of five . . . you doctors . . . every time you do not know what to do, you make a diagnosis of a virus or a psychosomatic pain".

I breathe deeply. "You're angry", I say. "It must be so frustrating; we have tried different kinds of solutions with no success. I am frustrated too. I am sorry I couldn't help you more so far".

His body softens, his breathing gets calmer when he says, "Yeah. . . . It is frustrating . . . No one can help and no one can help my father either . . . He is dying . . . ALS". He bows his head and whispers, "We are waiting for his death . . . there's nothing we can do".

"I am so sorry to hear about it", I say and sadness spreads in me when we look at each other in stillness.

His body suddenly stiffens and his painful eyes become indignant again. "Well, it doesn't matter now", he breaks the silence and his voice hardens. "I don't care about that, I don't even visit him".

I look at him, fighting his emotions, every tightened muscle in his body takes part in the effort, and sorrow expands in me.

"So you are about to lose your father", I say sotto voce.

Silence.

He bends his back and bows his head, his muscles are all contracted, he looks aching and suffering while his vitality wanes.

"Your muscles are all contracted when we talk about your father", I mention. "You're aching, aren't you?"

He nods, crouched in his chair with a twitch of pain in his face, looking at me with agonised eyes. "Look at me", he asks. "That's exactly how my father sat a few months ago in his armchair, droopy and bent. And now . . . now he cannot even do that, his muscles are too weak".

He stops talking, gazing at me with a shimmer of sadness in his eyes, surprised at his own words.

"So, your father's muscles can no longer hold him", I add and the sorrow in his eyes deepens. I hesitate, but then say it: "Rob, your father does not need you to contract your muscles for him, I think he would rather have your love".

His body softens, his muscles are more relaxed, his voice quavers when he says, "I miss him so much".

It has been three months since then. The intensity of his pain has diminished. "This pain is like a psychic barometer", he explained in one of our encounters. "Every time it comes back, I know I have to slow down".

And here he is again three months later.

"My father died last week", he says sadly.

"I am sorry", I say, "and, how are you?"

"I was able to be with him and hold his hand", he shares with me. "It wasn't easy, you know . . . my muscles ache . . . but it is OK, sometimes the body needs to bear the burden".

We are such a complicated organism, and our systems are deeply interconnected: our thinking patterns, our emotional life, our immune system, muscular system, our social network—any medical complaint, symptom or illness encompasses bodily, emotional, and cognitive aspects which constitute the human experience of our patient. In the previous chapter we have discussed the way symptoms and diseases need not be categorised as somatic or psychological, but instead seen as an expression of a broader experience. We have demonstrated how approaching our patients' experiences, requires us not only to listen to the content of the conversation and take biopsychosocial anamnesis, but to also attend to non-verbal language. We have reviewed various mechanisms in which the body speaks the psyche, and exemplified the magnitude of listening to the body's language in clinical practice.

In his seminal book *Emotional Intelligence*, Daniel Goldman (1996) proposes that more than 90% of our emotional experience is communicated nonverbally. While most of us are used to pay attention to the verbal content of our patients' stories regarding their bodies and lives, research has shown that by observing people's body language we learn much more about their experience than by asking them questions directly (Glawell, 2005; Knapp & Hall, 2010; Reich, 1967). Most of patients do not share relevant feelings such as fears, expectations, and thoughts regarding their medical complaint with their doctors even when asked directly. Patients might feel ashamed or unaware of their emotions. Studies in medical practice show that tuning into the body's language has significant effects on patient satisfaction, health outcomes, and malpractice claims (Riess & Kraft-Todd, 2014).

Even though most human interaction and communication is nonverbal, these kinds of communication skills are not ordinarily taught in courses where doctors learn to take medical histories, explain medical interventions, or deliver bad news. This spotlight on verbal communication might discount the fundamental role nonverbal cues have in the communication of emotions, symptoms, and illness. We are not properly prepared to enter an efficient dialogue without those skills.

Moreover, as already demonstrated in the previous chapter, symptoms and diseases might hold various meanings and communicate psychological pain and trauma. That means that together with listening nonverbal cues as a part of communication between doctors and patient, we also make room for the symptom and the illness as communicators of a broader experience, and seek for an integration of the mind and body in order to access a richer and more salient experience.

Rob's muscle pains constitute a part of a whole experience which is expressed in both verbal and nonverbal language. We believe that he attempted to identify and 'hurt on his father's behalf' without doing so consciously. But our interpretation is not what matters, interesting as it might be. Rob was able to attribute meaning to his pain, and it directly resulted in an improvement of his complaints. Throughout our encounter, his experience has changed and has been articulated in both languages. Attunement to his 'here and now' experience whilst listening to both languages has led to deeper connection with Rob, improved communication and a wider understanding of his symptom. Joined together, these qualities laid the ground for the whole experience to unfold overcoming the split between the bodily symptom and its psychological aspect. It was neither his body that improved nor his mind that was fixed; it was Rob who felt better—more present, more able to deal with the situations ahead.

In this chapter we will represent and demonstrate some practical skills for listening to the language of the body. Some of the skills can be easily implemented in clinical practice, and some need further training before putting in practice. We believe that incorporating these skills in medical practice would benefit clinical encounters significantly. We further wish to encourage you to find a local course which will provide practical and clinical tools for listening to the language of the body.

14.1 Tracking: Listening to the Patient's Body

Tracking is the skill of paying attention, as an active witness, to outward physical signs of our patients' present-moment experience (Kurtz, 1990; Martin, 2015). This type of attention was deeply explored in body psychotherapy from the days of Reich (1973, 1979) and the generations that followed—Alexander Lowen (1958, 1975); Gerda Boyesen (1980); David Boadella (1985, 1987) to mention a few. This type of listening and observing incorporate a curiosity about nonverbal indicators that pave the road into the internal experience of our patients and shed light on it. We track for nonverbal indicators such as: patient's breathing, body movements, gestures, postures, facial expressions, eye contact, and tone of voice (Ekman & Rosenberg, 2005; Marlock & Weiss, 2006; Martin, 2015).

Breathing is one of the most constant forms of our life, and yet at the same time it is dynamic and changing. It is a sensitive indicator of blood oxygenation, cardiac output, lung function, and a variety of other systemic medical conditions, and therefore observing our patients' breathing and listening to their lungs are fundamental in any routine physical examination. However, breathing patterns also express particular emotional positions and are directly affected by our level of stress and anxiety (Gilbert, 1999; Ogden et al., 2006; Rolef Ben-Shahar, 2014). When people are emotionally activated their breathing changes. It might become deep or shallow, fast or slow, centred more in the chest or belly and so on (Hendricks, 1995; Painter, 1984).

Eye contact is a key component of social cognition and is usually one of the first signs that one person has been noticed by another (Siegel, 1999). The quality of the eye contact and the patient's gaze gives us information regarding our engagement with our patient and his inner experience (e.g., absence of eye contact, pleading eyes, moist eyes, etc.) (Ziehl, 2000).

Facial expression is another substantial component of nonverbal communication. Several universal facial expressions were depicted in literature (Ekman & Friesen, 1969), and the ability to unravel them provides us with a valuable glance into our patient's experience and enhances empathic communication (Carr et al., 2003).

Posture is a powerful signal of our patients' emotions (Aviezer et al., 2012; Keleman, 1985; Painter, 1984). Stress and various emotions are all expressed in muscular changes, some of them are chronic and others are dynamic (e.g., contracted shoulders, straitening up, bending, etc.)

Tone of voice offers us important indicators regarding our patient's inner experience too. Cues such as intonation, intensity, loudness, and speed are all important to track (Martin, 2015).

Let us return to Rob and delve into his body language in the presented medical encounter. The descriptions below naturally stem from my interpretation and understanding of body language, and are not objective. However, as we hope to have demonstrated, our subjective experience of the other person—and our educated observation—provide us with rich information which could complement other data.

When Rob comes in with his medical complaint, his *pleading eyes* and *beseeching gaze* (eye contact, facial expression) reveal his neediness and helplessness. Afterwards, when I tell him there is no need for further blood tests, we can observe that *his begging eyes widely open* and his look is *penetrating and incensed* (eye contact, facial expression), his breathing gets deeper* (breathing*), *he straightens up* (posture) and *he raises his voice* (tone of voice). Paying attention to these nonverbal indicators enables me to engage with his inner experience of anger and frustration. Following this act of recognition and validation of his experience his body *softens* (posture), and *his breathing gets calmer* (breathing), indicating that we are reconnecting and he feels seen and understood. Sharing his father's terminal illness with me, he *bows his head* (posture) and *whispers* (tone of voice), letting me in to his sadness, pain, and sorrow. When *his soften body suddenly stiffens* (posture), *his painful eyes become indignant again* (eye contact, facial expression), and *his voice hardens* (tone of voice), I can see how he is fighting his emotions, and how every tightened muscle in his body takes part in the effort. His symptom of muscle pain is then enlivened in our meeting when *he bends his back and bows his head, his muscles are all contracted, he looks aching and suffering while his vitality wanes,* transforming the original medical complaint into a richer and more salient experience, ensuing an integration of mind and body.

As we can see, tracking allows us to notice the inner experience of our patients more deeply without asking unnecessary questions or waiting for the patient to disclose. It is an act of being interested in inhabiting the patient's experience and listening deeply to body and emotions. In other words, we are curious not only about the story that the patient is telling us, but also about the storyteller. Who is telling us about his illness or symptoms? Is he an anxious father worrying about his daughter's fever? Is she a frustrated woman with chronic low back pain?

When this kind of attunement is conducted in the light of empathic and compassionate human presence it enhances empathy (Finlay, 2006) and might guide us to a more accurate diagnosis and more suitable interventions. It might be worthwhile to mention that we are biologically wired to listen like that—this is no rocket science. The main difference between intuitive nonverbal listening to the one demonstrated above is cultivation: honing skills of nonverbal listening through training and ongoing practice.

14.2 Bodily Resonance: Listening to Our Own Body

It is not only our patients' bodies that communicate clearly about them; it is our body as well. Our own body is also constantly communicating data regarding the mutual experience with our patients as we resonate with them. Chapter 10 explored the role of mirror neurons, exemplifying how emotional bodily resonance systems are the substrate for emotional intelligence that allows us to feel the other through our own bodies by breaking the walls between us.

The capacity to sense the other through our own body is a natural and innately human. Resonance describes a primarily nonverbal and affective response to what is happening in the other. It is a conversation taking place in an unmediated fashion between bodies (Rolef Ben-Shahar, 2014). For example, when a depressed patient enters the clinic, we oftentimes feel tired and depleted of vital energy. On the other hand, when an angry patient comes in, we might feel the vigilance and tension within ourselves.

Being aware of our changing body sensations, as these are affected by the presence of our patients, could endow us with information not only about ourselves but also about our patients' experience. In other words, our bodily sensations, the way we breath, how we make eye contact with our patient, and our posture are all affected by the interaction with our patient. In the same way we track our patients' nonverbal language, being mindful to ours could prove a valuable skill.

The interaction with Rob exemplifies how not only tracking his bodily language is important, but also the awareness of the doctor's body. When he expresses his helplessness, my *body draws back and shrinks*; when he shares his father's illness, *sadness spreads in me*. These two examples demonstrate how our bodies communicate with our patients', how they affect each other, how they hold essential information about the 'here and now' experience of the patient, and how the process of resonance constitutes a pulsatile ongoing platform for embodied empathy (Finlay, 2006; Rudebeck, 2000).

14.3 Listening to the Symptom

As physicians, we are used to listening to symptoms either by taking medical history and asking about the duration, intensity, precipitating and alleviating factors, or by means of physical examination. When patients decide to see a doctor, they have to choose how to convey their symptoms in the medical encounter. Some symptoms might be clear and unequivocal, whereas others are much more complex or opaque to put into words. Patients reveal diverse ways of coding their messages by using indirect forms of communication. When patients communicate personal distress through bodily symptoms, they express aspects of their illness experience that can be easily accessible in words (Freeman, 2016).

Rudebeck (2000) accentuates the importance of engaging with the patient's experience of a symptom as part of a diagnostic process. He writes: "A medical diagnosis is always made in two steps. . . . The first is about grasping the experience presented by the patient, and the second about interpreting the experience the way it has been grasped. Often, but far from exclusively, the interpretation will be made within the biomedical frame of reference. The first diagnostic step rests on intersubjectivity, and the second on a striving for objectivity. The better the doctor's comprehension fits with what the patient actually is experiencing, the more plausible it is that the diagnostic judgement will be accurate" (p. 5).

By tracking the patient's bodily language and being mindful to bodily resonance we can better grasp the experience of the symptom that the patient presents. We would like to suggest two questions that may help us attune and listen to the symptoms in ways that could deepen and expand our understanding of symptoms:

1.   How does the patient feel about his symptom?

Patients develop various kinds of feelings towards their symptoms. They might be afraid, angry, frustrated, despaired, disconnected, or sometimes even relieved. We can reveal those feelings by being attentive to nonverbal communication or by asking direct questions. Rob's feelings of helplessness, frustration, and anger expressed mostly nonverbally, constitute an integral part of his experience. Ignoring these feelings could have had deleterious influence on the medical encounter (and hamper diagnosis). Collaborating with his affective experience in an empathic way cultivated the therapeutic alliance and facilitated the ensuing process of understanding the symptom as a part of a whole experience.

2.   What could the symptom be conveying? Seeking the symptom's attributed meaning. What is the symptom telling me about the patient's body and mind?

By gathering and integrating verbal and nonverbal information referring to the experience of the symptom, together with our medical objective knowledge, we can try to answer these questions. Frequently, patients (and doctors) are unable to make the linkage between their emotions and bodily symptoms. Oftentimes the connection and understanding are accessible, while sometimes it is impassable (Freeman, 2016). Rob's fighting against his emotions towards his father's suffering by tightening his muscles, became a point where body and mind reconnected, where cognitive, emotional, and somatic aspects of the whole experience reunited and meaning unfolded.

This kind of process can be enhanced by attuning to nonverbal language such as tracking and resonance and by other skills that cultivate the connection of body and mind such as mindfulness, focusing, drawing, and writing (Lin & Payne, 2014).

While these skills might be valuable in medical encounter, in order to use them skilfully in clinical practice doctors need further training and practice, which is beyond the scope of this book.

In summary, contact with our patients' experience means making room for the concrete and symbolic ways their body speaks. As Westland (2015) beautifully writes: "The body is the source of nonverbal communication-a distracted gaze and slumped shoulders. A lively look in the eyes, or animated hand gestures. We can all see and come to understand this kind of communication through learning how to read our internal body sensations (including our intuitions) and couple them with our observations" (p. 2).

References

Aviezer, H., Trope, Y., & Todorov, A. (2012). Holistic person processing: Faces with bodies tell the whole story. *Journal of Personality and Social Psychology, 103*, 20–37.

Boadella, D. (1985). *Wilhelm Reich: The evolution of his work*. London: Arkana.

Boadella, D. (1987). *Lifestreams: An introduction to biosynthesis*. London: Routledge & Kegan Paul.

Boyesen, G. (Ed.). (1980). *Collected papers on biodynamic psychology*. London: Biodynamic Psychology Publications.

Carr, L., Iacoboni, M., Dubeau, M.C., Mazziotta, J.C., & Lenzi, G.L. (2003). Neural mechanisms of empathy in humans: A relay from neural systems for imitation to limbic areas. *Proceedings of the National Academy of Sciences of the U S A., 100*, 5497–5502.

Ekman, P., & Friesen, W.V. (1969). The repertoire of nonverbal behavior: Categories, origins, usage, and coding. *Semiotica, 1*, 49–98.

Ekman, P., & Rosenberg, E.L. (Eds.). (2005). *What the face reveals: Basic and applied studies of spontaneous expression using the facial action coding system*. New York, NY: Oxford University Press.

Finlay, L. (2006). The body's disclosure in phenomenological research. *Qualitative Research in Psychology, 3*(19–30).

Freeman, T.R. (2016). *McWhinney's textbook of family medicine*. Oxford: Oxford University Press.

Gilbert, C. (1999). Breathing: The legacy of Wilhelm Reich. *Journal of Bodywork & Movement Therapies, 3*(2), 97–106.

Glawell, M. (2005). *Blink*. New York, NY: Little, Brown.

Goldman, D. (1996). *Emotional intelligence: Why can it matter more than IQ*. New York, NY: Bantam Books.

Hendricks, G. (1995). *Conscious breathing: Breathwork for health, stress release, and personal mastery*. New York, NY: Bantam Books.

Keleman, S. (1985). *Emotional anatomy*. Berkley, CA: Center Press.

Knapp, M.L., & Hall, J.A. (2010). *Nonverbal communication in human interaction* (7th ed.). Boston, MA: Wadsworth, Cengage Learning.

Kurtz, R. (1990). *Body-centered psychotherapy: The Hakomi method*. Mendocino, CA: Life-Rhythm.

Lin, Y., & Payne, H. (2014). The BodyMind approach, medically unexplained symptoms and personal construct psychology. *International Journal for Body, Movement and Dance in Psychotherapy, 9*(3), 154–166.

Lowen, A. (1958). *The language of the body*. New York, NY: Macmillan Publishing.

Lowen, A. (1975). *Bioenergetics*. New York, NY: Arkana.

Marlock, G., & Weiss, H. (Eds.). (2006). *Handbook of body psychotherapy*. Stuttgart: Schattauer.

Martin, D. (2015). The skills of tracking and contact. In H. Weiss, G. Johanson, & L. Monda (Eds.), *Hakomi mindfulness-centered somatic psychotherapy: A comprehensive guide to theory and practice*. New York, NY: W.W. Norton & Co.

Ogden, P., Minton, K., & Pain, C. (2006). *Trauma and the body: A sensorimotor approach to psychotherapy*. New York, NY: W.W. Norton & Co.

Painter, J.W. (1984). *Deep bodywork and personal development*. Mill Valley, CA: Bodymind Books.

Reich, W. (1967). *Reich speaks of Freud*. Harmondsworth, London: Penguin.

Reich, W. (1973). *The function of the orgasm* (V.R. Carfagno, Trans.). London: Souvenir Press.

Reich, W. (1979). *Selected writing*. New York, NY: Farrar, Straus & Giroux.

Riess, H., & Kraft-Todd, G. (2014). E.M.P.A.T.H.Y.: A tool to enhance nonverbal communication between clinicians and their patients. *Academic Medicine, 89*, 1108–1112.

Rolef Ben-Shahar, A. (2014). *Touching the relational edge: Body psychotherapy*. London: Karnac Books.

Rudebeck, C.E. (2000). The doctor, the patient and the body. *Scandinavian Journal of Health Care, 18*, 4–8.

Siegel, D.J. (1999). *The developing mind: Toward a neurobiology of interpersonal experience*. New York, NY: Guilford Press.

Westland, G. (2015). *Verbal and non-verbal communication in psychotherapy*. New York, NY: W.W. Norton & Co.

Ziehl, S. (2000). *Character structure: Integrating Reichian and post-Reichian perspectives*. Paper presented at the Deep Bodywork Training Material.

15 Doctor-Patient Communication

A Dialogue Between Bodies and Minds

Incidentally, it's easy to write prescriptions, but difficult to come to an understanding with people.

—Franz Kafka, "A Country Doctor", 1917

Judy has not been sleeping for a few weeks. She gets into bed and all these bothering thoughts intrude, thwarting any chance of falling asleep. She cannot talk about it with anyone, not her husband, not her friends, no one. She is so afraid. She cannot even think about it. She works day and night so she will have no time to think about it.

It all started a month ago. At first, she thought there is nothing to worry about. But when her low back pain refused to go away, she became more and more concerned. It hurts day and night; sometimes she takes NSAIDS with a partial relief. She cannot even think about the option that her cancer is back. It cannot be; she cannot go through chemotherapy again.

She has considered going to Dr. Jones a few times. She has even made an appointment and cancelled. Imagining his perturbed eyes looking at her after telling him about her aching back, she felt as if the sword of death is penetrating her heart. After thinking it over time and again, she has decided. She would ask for sleeping pills. At least she will not spend the rest of her short life without sleeping.

He is in the middle of a busy day, when Judy comes in. He has been her family doctor in the past few years. She is a forty-seven-year-old brilliant business woman. Three years ago, he diagnosed a breast lump, a month later she had mastectomy and started chemotherapy. Everything went well with no exceptional complications. He has not seen her for a few months. She gets into his office in a hurry looking a bit upset and tired. "I've come to ask for prescription for sleeping pills", she says, "That's all", she smiles anxiously.

"Please, sit down, Judy", he asks her. "I would like to hear more".

"Well, there's nothing to tell. I just want to sleep better at night. That's all. So, could you please give me some pills? It's not a problem, isn't it?" she asks impatiently. "It's only a prescription."

"It is not a problem, but I do have to ask you some questions", he replies.

"What questions?" she asks reluctantly.

"How long have you had difficulty with your sleep? Is it hard to fall asleep or do you wake during the night?" he asks.

"All these questions . . . why is everything so complicated?" she raises her voice. "I am in a hurry and I really don't like being here, so why making it harder?"

Trying to control his restlessness and grumpiness he says," I need to hear more about your sleeping habits before I prescribe you pills".

Doctor- patient communication constitutes an integral part of any medical encounter. It has an extensive impact on the course of the encounter and the effectiveness of the treatment (Begum, 2014; Shukla et al., 2010). It is essential for the evolution of meaningful and trustworthy relationship between the doctors and patients, enhancing doctors' diagnostic capability, managing difficult clinical encounters, improving compliance, health outcomes, and patients' satisfaction, ameliorating clinicians' satisfaction and decreasing work stress (Begum, 2014; Ranjan et al., 2015; Shukla et al., 2010).

Despite the well appreciated benefits of good doctor-patient communication, studies demonstrate patient discontent even when doctors consider the communication adequate (Stewart, 1995). Mentioned barriers to effective communication include: lack of insight due to inadequate knowledge and training in communication skills, unnoticed non-verbal components, and human limitations derived from an overburdened setting (Ranjan et al., 2015).

While patients come to their doctors with various expectations, fears, concerns, and health beliefs, they often have difficulty in fully expressing these issues with their doctors. As a result, some issues might go unvoiced, be introduced in a "by the way" presentation at the end of the consultation or expressed implicitly in other ways. In other words, the way by which patients present their agendas may not reflect their perceived importance or match the doctor's prioritisation (Hamilton & Britten, 2006).

Campion et al. (1992) depicted three principal agenda types (physical, emotional, and social) presented in medical interview. In their research, they found that both doctor and patient address physical agendas to a similar high degree, whereas patients present emotional agendas to a far greater extent than doctors address these concerns. In a qualitative research investigating unvoiced patients' agendas (Barry et al., 2000), agenda items most commonly voiced were symptoms and requests for diagnoses and prescriptions, while most common unvoiced agenda items related to worries, patients' ideas about what was wrong, side effects, reluctance to prescriptions, and information regarding social context. Agenda items that were not advertised in the medical encounter engendered specific problematic outcomes, unwanted prescriptions, non-use of prescriptions, and non-adherence to treatment. The gap between both agendas may negatively affect treatment decisions and therefore influence patients' outcomes (Ha et al., 2010). Judy's 'simple' request for sleeping pills masks a more complex agenda. If left unvoiced, outcome will be affected.

How can we facilitate patients to reveal fuller agendas?

In this chapter we will review and discuss known communicative skills, and try to expand them by interweaving concepts, proficiencies, and body of knowledge introduced in the previous chapters. We believe that integrating these issues can upgrade doctor-patient communication in clinical practice.

15.1 The Medical Interview

The medical interview provides the context for taking the patient's history, collecting relevant biopsychosocial information regarding the problem and reaching understanding of the patient's experience and agenda. Whether interviewing has the purpose of history taking, consultation, or breaking bad news, it is a process of both verbal and nonverbal communication that holds three main goals: generating a good interpersonal relationship, facilitating a mutual exchange of information, and fostering shared decision making (Arora, 2003; Boon & Stewart, 1998; Bredart et al., 2005).

Collaborative communication lays on a dynamic relationship involving a two-way exchange of information (both verbal and nonverbal). A fruitful information exchange enables the elicitation and exploration of hidden components of the patient's agenda, thus facilitating shared decision making (Arora, 2003; Ha et al., 2010; Lee et al., 2002; Minhas, 2007).

When Judy comes to her doctor with an explicit agenda for sleeping pills, she conceals her "real story". Unravelling the hidden agenda might have critical consequences on her health.

Throughout the medical encounter, it is essential to recognise patient's expectations, emotions, wishes, barriers and benefits of treatment, functional and symbolic meaning of disease (Ha et al., 2010). Enabling patients to express their emotions and concerns, and engaging with the patient's experience (see previous chapters) is of paramount importance for improving the quality of care and health outcomes (Arora, 2003; Diette & Rand, 2007). Our capacity to understand our patients' whole experience, and communicate that understanding with empathy is crucial.

How can we enhance a collaborative communication?

15.2 Two-Way Communication

Doctor-patient communication is an interactive discourse between minds and bodies, wherein simultaneously with the exchange on the verbal level, both patients and doctors influence each other's affect, arousal, and body language. As discussed in chapter 10, mirror neurons research provides a neurobiological understanding of emotional bodily resonance systems which allow us to feel the other through our own and affect each other. Subsequent studies illustrated interconnected and associative neural circuits that endue shared emotional experiences between an observer and the observed person (Adolphs, 2009). Porge's (2011) polyvagal theory presents a third neural circuit regulating autonomic nervous system which forms a functional "social engagement system" (see chapter 2). This theory emphasises the significance of social relationships when facing overwhelming emotions and stress. It explains why a kind face or a soothing tone of voice can dramatically alter the way we feel, and why attunement with another person can shift us out of stressful states.

As previously mentioned, resonance represents a primarily nonverbal and affective response to what is happening in the other. It is described as a conversation taking place in an unmediated fashion between bodies. Just as our bodily sensations and emotions are all affected by the interaction with our patients, so do ours affect our patients. Meaning that when we are resourced, mindful, attuned, self-regulated, empathic, and compassionate, we are better capable of regulating our patients' intense affect and overwhelming emotions. Therefore, our self-regulatory capacity within the relational context of the medical encounter is of paramount importance in the interaction between doctors and patients. When we comprehend that beneficial communication rests on a dynamic process between bodies and minds, our presence and the relationship become an impactful central axis that affects and regulates patients' bodies and minds.

When Judy is anxious and demanding, her doctor is affected—feeling restless and angry. This process might lead to reactive countertransference (see Chapter 9) and end in a clash between two agendas. Alternatively, her doctor might be mindful to his experience, regulate himself by connecting to his resources such as breathing or grounding (see Chapters 5, 6), and then his serenity and openness would be felt by Judy and probably would calm and soften her. Doctor-patient communication is a two-way interaction involving bi-directional verbal and nonverbal exchange of information. In this process we have to cultivate deep listening to the patient's verbal content and to his body language; we need to be mindful to our own experience; and we have to generate a facilitative response.

15.3 Active Listening

Active listening is an important communication skill for gaining relevant information regarding our patients' medical condition, understanding their experience, giving them permission to speak, and acknowledging their suffering (Fassaert et al., 2007). In the course of the medical encounter, worthy information is being articulated via verbal and nonverbal channels. Attentive listening to both channels of communication would assist doctors to understand patients' experience of illness, help recognise hidden agendas, enable patients to disclose related specific concerns and emotional content, reduce stress, increase shared decision, reinforce the healing process, and improve clinical outcomes (Jagosh et al., 2011; Wissow et al., 1994).

So, what should we listen to?

In the verbal aspect we should listen to both biomedical and psychosocial content. That means using open-ended questions that invite an open discussion and elicit a wide range of information about both medical issues and relevant social life. Open questions should comprise physical issues (e.g., "What can you tell me about your headache?"), social history (e.g., "Tell me about your work".), emotional and behavioural difficulties (e.g., "What concerns do you have?").

As doctors we frequently interrupt our patients. Studies show that the average time between the patient beginning to tell his story and the doctor's interruption is lies between 18 to 23 seconds (Beckman & Frankel, 1984; Marvel et al., 1999). A cross-sectional survey (Marvel et al., 1999) that examined the extent to which family physicians elicit the agenda of patients' concerns brought to the medical encounter showed that using open questions until a complete agenda would be identified, took 6 seconds longer than interviews in which the patient's agenda is interrupted. Active listening necessitates us to listen attentively, give the patient a chance to ponder, elaborate or clarify his problem without interrupting (Fassaert et al., 2007). In other words, we need to give patients time and space to present their problem, and allow them to finish talking. This kind of communication encourages patients to share ideas, cultivates the partnership between doctor and patient, and hence lays the foundation for mutual participation (Neo, 2011).

In the previous chapter we have discussed the importance of observing patients' body language. We have illustrated how much information about their experience we reveal by tracking our patients' body language and by being mindful to our bodies' sensations and feelings (bodily resonance). Active listening encompasses listening to emotions, affect, and the body. In other words, we listen to more than just the verbal story the patient is telling us, but also to the storyteller's experience. The indicators of our patients' experience are mostly nonverbal (Goldman, 1996), and research has shown that by observing people's body language we learn much more about their experience than by asking them questions directly (Glawell, 2005; Knapp & Hall, 2010). Tracking nonverbal cues might be a critical entry point when patients do not share relevant feelings such as fears, expectations, and thoughts regarding their medical complaint or disagreements with medical interventions when directly asked (Glawell, 2005; Knapp & Hall, 2010; Riess & Kraft-Todd, 2014). Our own body is also constantly communicating information about the mutual experience with our patients as we resonate limbically with them (see previous chapter). In other words, when communicating with a patient, paying attention to our bodily sensations, affect, changes in posture, eye contact, and other bodily indicators endow us with valuable information about transference dynamics (see chapter 9) and the patient's experience. If Judy's doctor becomes mindful of his grumpiness and restlessness upon facing her demand for a sleeping pills prescription, and is able to perceive his feelings as information regarding their interaction and Judy's inner stressful experience, he will be better able to choose how to respond instead of reacting to her insistence in an unwanted way.

15.4 Facilitative Response

After listening deeply to our patient and getting the picture of the nature and meaning of his/her experience, communicating that understanding and engaging with our patient's experience with empathy and compassion is essential. In chapters 10 and 11 we have introduced the qualities of human presence, empathy, and compassion in medical care, elaborated on their beneficial effects for both patients and doctors, and discussed ways of implementing them in daily practice. Our affective presence and responsiveness have powerful impact on the quality of the medical encounter. There are substantial variations in doctors' responsiveness to patients, depending on their communicative skills, context, momentary state of mind, and personal issues.

Just as empathy is communicated through both verbal and nonverbal behaviours (see chapters 10 and 11), so is a facilitative response.

Literature has shown that through nonverbal behaviours, patients get an indication of their doctor's care, attention, respect, understanding, and affiliation with them (Davis & Fallowfield, 1991; Gallagher et al., 2005; Kraft-Todd et al., 2017; Riess & Kraft-Todd, 2014; Suchman et al., 1997). The most refined and subtle signals and cues of our nonverbal attitude are detected in the amygdala much faster than the prefrontal cortex's capability of processing verbal content. That is, nonverbal language is not only processed faster, but also has more influential effect than verbal statements (Adams et al., 2003; Birdwhistell, 1970; Phillips et al., 2003).

Given the significance of our nonverbal approach as doctors, we need to be aware of both our patients' nonverbal indicators and our own nonverbal behaviour. We should be mindful of the implications of our body language and use it as another communicative platform (Kraft-Todd et al., 2017; Riess & Kraft-Todd, 2014). Doctors' nonverbal behaviours and gestures considerably influence patients' perceptions of their doctors' empathy and doctor-patient collaboration (Montague et al., 2013; Riess & Kraft-Todd, 2014; Roter & Hall, 2006). Meaningful eye contact (especially when using the computer during the medical encounter) and facial expressions are crucial elements for engaging with patients. Posture has significant effect too. For instance, an open body posture (uncrossed arms) and sitting position at eye level with patients convey mutual respect, openness, and interest in the patient's experience (Kraft-Todd et al., 2017; Riess & Kraft-Todd, 2014). When we are mindful of our body language, we are capable of choosing other ways of bodily interaction which would facilitate a better response and cultivate collaborative communication.

As already mentioned, a facilitative response has both verbal and nonverbal aspects. In the verbal aspect, successful information exchange in the medical encounter should be communicated in a simple and direct manner, avoiding the use of medical jargons, enabling patients to respond and engage in a mutual discussion (Neo, 2011). Another important aspect is making verbal contact with the patient's present experience. Naming the patient's affect lets the patient know that his doctor is listening to him; he is interested nonjudgmentally in his mental state; and he understands his feelings and experience (Martin, 2015; Riess & Kraft-Todd, 2014). When Judy's doctor observes her anger, anxiety, frustration, and tiredness, he can make a few verbal contacts with her experience such as: "You look angry", "You must be exhausted", or "It must be frustrating". In other words, through tracking (see previous chapter) and by being mindful of our patient's affect, we can verbally address a relevant aspect of his experience.

Let's go back now to Judy and her doctor.

He notices her clenched lips, her contracted shoulders, and her leg moving nervously after he asks to hear more about her sleeping habits (listening to patient's body language). *His breathing gets heavier and he leans back while looking at her* (self-awareness of own body sensations and posture). *He takes a deep breath* (resourcing), *leans forward to her* (facilitative nonverbal response), *and says, "You must be exhausted"* (making verbal contact with her experience).

"I am", she says and her body softens, sadness blended with anxiety in her eyes (listening to patient's body language).

"You look worried (verbal contact), *what is it* (open question regarding emotional content)?"

She breathes deeply, her head down when she whispers, "I am afraid . . . I have this low back pain for weeks. That's why I can't sleep".

"Afraid cancer is back?" he asks softly (hidden agenda revealed).

Silence in the room. He looks at her, she looks so fragile, and his heart fills with compassion. They breathe deeply together, looking at each other's eyes in a precious moment of connectedness.

References

Adams, R.B. Jr., Gordon, H.L., Baird, A.A., Ambady, N., & Kleck, R.E. (2003). Effects of gaze on amygdala sensitivity to anger and fear faces. *Science, 300*, 1536.

Adolphs, R. (2009). The social brain: Neural basis of social knowledge. *Annual Review Psychology, 60*, 693–716.

Arora, N. (2003). Interacting with cancer patients: The significance of physicians' communication behavior. *Social Science and Medicine, 57*(5), 791–806.

Barry, C.A., Bradley, C.P., Britten, N., Stevenson, F.A., & Barber N. (2000). Patients' unvoiced agendas in general practice consultations: Qualitative study. *British Medical Journal, 320*(7244), 1246–1250.

Beckman, H.B., & Frankel, R.N. (1984). The effect of physician behavior on the collection of data. *Annals of Internal Medicine, 101*, 682.

Begum, T. (2014). Doctor patient communication: A review. *Journal of Bangladesh College of Physicians and Surgeons, 32*(2), 84–88.

Birdwhistell, R.L. (1970). *Kinesics and context: Essays on body motion communication.* Philadelphia, PA: University of Pennsylvania Press.

Boon, H., & Stewart, M. (1998). Patient-physician communication assessment instrument: 1986 to 1996 in review. *Patient Education and Counseling, 35*, 161–76.

Bredart, A., Bouleuc, C., & Dolbeault, S. (2005). Doctor-patient communication and satisfaction with care in oncology. *Current Opinion in Oncology, 17*(14), 351–354.

Campion, P.D., Butler, N.M., & Cox, A.D. (1992). Principle agendas of doctors and patients in general practice consultations. *Family Practice, 9*, 181–190.

Davis, H., & Fallowfield, L. (1991). Counselling and communication in health care: The current situation. In H. Davis & L. Fallowfield (Eds.), *Counselling and communication in health care*. Chichester, West Sussex: Wiley.

Diette, G.B., & Rand, C. (2007). The contributing role of health-care communication to health disparities for minority patients with asthma. *Chest, 135*(5 supplement), 802S-809S.

Fassaert, T., van Dulmen, S., Schellevis, F., & Bensing, J. (2007). Active listening in medical consultations: Development of the Active Listening Observation Scale (ALOS-global). *Patient Education and Counseling, 68*(3), 258–264.

Gallagher, T.J., Hartung, P.J., Gerzina, H., Gergory, S.W. Jr, & Merolla, D. (2005). Further analysis of a doctor-patient nonverbal communication instrument. *Patient Education and Counseling, 57*, 262–271.

Ha, J.F., Anat, D.S., & Longnecker, N. (2010). Doctor-patient communication: A review. *The Ochsner Journal, 10*, 38–43.

Hamilton, W., & Britten, N. (2006). Patient agendas in primary care. *British Medical Journal, 332*, 1225.

Jagosh J., Boudreau J.D., Steinert Y., MacDonald M.E., & Ingram L. (2011). The importance of physician listening from the patients' perspective: Enhancing diagnosis, healing and the doctor-patient relationship. *Patient Education and Counseling, 85*(3), 369–374.

Kraft-Todd, G.T., Reinero, D.A., Kelley, J.M., Heberlein, A.S., Baer, L., & Riess, H. (2017). Empathic nonverbal behavior increases ratings of both warmth and competence in a medical context. *PLoS One, 12*(5), 1–16.

Lee, S.J., Back, A.L., Block, S.D., & Stewart, S.K. (2002). Enhancing physician-patient communication. *Hematology American Society Hematologic Education Program, 1*, 464–483.

Martin, D. (2015). The skills of tracking and contact. In H. Weiss, G. Johanson, & L. Monda (Eds.), *Hakomi mindfulness-centered somatic psychotherapy: A comprehensive guide to theory and practice*. New York, NY: W.W. Norton & Co.

Marvel, M.K., Epstein, R.M., Flowers, K., & Beckman, H.B. (1999). Soliciting the patient's agenda: Have we improved? *Journal of the American Medical Association, 281*(3), 283–287.

Minhas, R. (2007). Does copying clinical or sharing correspondence to patient result in better care? *International Journal of Clinical Practice, 61*(8), 1390–1395.

Montague, E., Chen, P-Y., Xu, J., Chewning, B., & Barrett, B. (2013). Nonverbal interpersonal interactions in clinical encounters and patient perceptions of empathy. *Journal of Participatory Medicine, 5*, e33.

Neo, L.F. (2011). Working toward the best doctor-patient communication. *Singapore Medical Journal, 52*(10), 720–725.

Phillips, M.L., Drevets, W.C., Rauch, S.L., & Lane, R. (2003). Neurobiology of emotion perception I: The neural basis of normal emotion perception. *Biological Psychiatry, 54*, 504–514.

Porges, S.W. (2011). *The Polyvagal theory: Neurophysiological foundations of emotions, attachment, communication, and self-regulation.* New York, NY: W.W. Norton & Co.

Ranjan, P., Kumari, A., & Chakrawarty, A. (2015). How can doctors improve their communication skills? *Journal of Clinical and Diagnostic Research, 9*(3), JE01-JE04.

Riess, H., & Kraft-Todd, G. (2014). E.M.P.A.T.H.Y.: A tool to enhance nonverbal communication between clinicians and their patients. *Academic Medicine, 89*(8), 1108–1112.

Roter, D.L., & Hall, J.A. (2006). *Doctors talking with patients/patients talking with doctors: Improving communication in medical visits* (2nd ed.). Westport, CT: Praeger Publishers.

Shukla, A.K., Yadav, V.S., & Kastury, N. (2010). Doctor-patient communication: An important but often ignored aspect in clinical medicine. *Journal, Indian Academy of Clinical Medicine, 11*, 208–211.

Stewart, M.A. (1995). Effective physician-patient communication and health outcomes: A review. *Canadian Medical Association Journal, 152*(9), 1423–1433.

Suchman, A.L., Markakis, K., Beckman, H.B., & Frankel, R. (1997). A model of empathic communication in the medical interview. *Journal of American Medical Association, 277*(8), 678–682.

Wissow, L.S., Roter, D.L., & Wilson, M.E. (1994). Pediatrician interview style and mothers' disclosure of psychosocial issues. *Pediatrics, 9*, 289–295.

16 Practical Body-Mind Interventions in Medical Care

Throughout the book, we have presented a body of research that exemplifies the complex interaction between body and mind and endeavoured to encourage a broadening of the diagnostic lens, to include emotional, cognitive, sociocultural, and other perspectives that influence the subjective experience of our patients (and our own), and thus contribute to the complete medical picture. In this chapter we will introduce you with practical body-mind interventions that based on our clinical experience and research might have a positive impact on a variety of medical conditions.

16.1 Chronic Pain

Emma is a fifty-year-old woman suffering from chronic low back pain for more than two years. Her back started to hurt after nursing her dying mother for a few months. Since then she has been disabled several times by excruciating sciatic pain. While MRI showed a mild disk bulge, she suffered debilitating pain and found it difficult to work as a hairdresser. When anti-inflammatory drugs and physiotherapy could hardly relieve her symptoms, Emma became more and more concerned and anxious regarding her deteriorating function, and developed mild depressive symptoms as well. Even when she started working in an administrative position, she could not sit for long time and soon found herself unemployed. She could realise that her anxiety and mild depression might aggravate her pain and decline her physical function, but it did little to lessen her misery.

Chronic pain imposes substantial challenges for people. Prevalence of chronic pain varies widely, with between 8% and 45% of the population reporting chronic pain, and between 10% and 15% of the population presenting to their general practitioner (McQuay & Moore, 2008). Chronic pain is associated with significant increase in morbidity and mortality (Torrance et al., 2010; Mäntyselkä et al., 2003) and co-morbid depression (Barnett et al., 2012).

Standard treatment for alleviation of pain is based on pharmacological therapy. These biomedical approaches may be unsatisfactory in breaking out of the cycle of chronic pain, and lack long-term benefit or subject these patients to several risks (Gatchel et al., 2014; Shariff et al., 2010)

The biopsychosocial approach depicts pain and disability as a complex and dynamic interplay made of physiological, psychological, and social factors that affect one another in the complexity of chronic pain (Gatchel et al., 2014).

Chronic pain management strategies include drug interventions, psychological approaches such as CBT, physiotherapy, peripheral nervous system stimulation, complementary medicine interventions, body-mind interventions, and self-management techniques (Mills et al., 2016; Sharif et al., 2010).

Self-management is defined as actions which augment function, improve mood, and alleviate pain by affecting emotional, cognitive, and behavioural responses to pain (Cameron, 2012). Medical research reports that self-management might be a valuable tool for attaining better outcomes in patients suffering from chronic pain (Astin, 2004). In their research, Shariff and her colleagues (2010) demonstrated that a sense of well-being in those coping with chronic pain could be better achieved through various mind-body self-management strategies. This management strategy is based on the recognition that body and mind do not function as isolated entities, and consist of techniques such as visualisation; breathing and mindfulness might help keep pain at a level that is compatible with functional life. These kinds of techniques have two important aspects. The first one refers to the possibility of noticing the pain and not reacting to it with emotions, urges, thoughts, and additional body sensations (McCracken et al., 2007).

There is a well-known talk attributed to the Buddha in which he describes a man that was shot with an arrow, and right afterward, he shot himself with another one (such as sorrow, anger, anxiety, self-flagellation, etc.), resulting in the pain of two arrows. This ancient understanding that the experience of physical pain is followed by an response of reluctance and suffering becomes possible by using body-mind techniques to enhance the possibility of waving the second arrow (Siegel, 2005). The second aspect of this strategy refers to improving the ability to live with the pain on an everyday basis and adapting activities in order to achieve a better life quality (Shariff et al., 2010). Unlike the attitude of trying to get rid of pain, in some of these techniques patients are instructed to focus on their pain instead of trying to avoid it. In several studies where subjects were exposed to ischemic pain produced by cold water or blocking blood circulation, those who were instructed to focus on their painful sensations reported significant reduction in their pain experience compared to those who were instructed to distract them from pain (Leventhal, 1984). These findings entail the realisation that focus on pain may be therapeutic, and give scientific rigor to body-mind interventions based on this principle.

We would like to introduce you with two practical techniques for self-management of acute and chronic pain that might be used in medical practice.

The Scale of Pain

This technique has extensive use in hypnotic therapies, while using altered states of consciousness (trance states), but since people suffering from pain are experiencing the world subjectively different to people without pain, it is a highly effective tool even without applying hypnotic skills. It is based on three assumptions: The first one regards to the fact that the mind and body are connected and can mutually impact each other, the second one relates to the presumption that we find it easier to believe that we can make things worse than to believe we can improve our conditions, and the third assumption concerns the associative transition from one modality of experience (pain, kinaesthetic) to another (visual) and back.

1. Ask the patient to identify the pain and focus on it. It might be useful to ask some sensory specific questions about the pain (sharp or dull, radiating or local, etc.).
2. Patient is requested to imagine (if they can visualise, that's good—but not necessary) a scale ranging between 1 and 10, where 1 indicates the most comfort and 10 the most severe pain. Ask the patient to imagine a needle showing where on the scale their pain is.
3. Ask the patient to very gently move the needle higher on the scale. If, for example, the needle shows 7, you can ask them to move the needle to 7.25, then 7.5. Take time to create a change that is not tormenting but can be experienced as more aversive. Please ensure you ask the patient to move the needle on the scale and not make the pain worse—we want to create a body-mind association between the visual and the pain experience.
4. Only then ask the patient, with every breath, to start bringing the scale down. Keep directing the patient to do so slowly. Only stopping when the pain has significantly decreased.
5. If the decreasing of pain slows down or stops, you can try increasing it again before repeating stage 4.

Most people can easily trust that they can influence their symptoms for the worse. The transition from kinaesthetic to visual processing, coupled with this belief, can support a pain-management technique that, if practiced, can not only help the physician but also be taken home by the client, implemented, and improved.

Thermal Pain Management Control

This technique works on similar principles to the scale of pain, and is more effective with highly visual people and children.

1. Ask the patient to identify the pain and focus on it. It might be useful to ask some sensory specific questions about the pain (sharp or dull, radiating or local, etc.).
2. Patient is requested to imagine a screen and a thermal picture of their body, where painful areas are marked by the red/orange palate shades, and comfortable parts are blue/greenish.

3. Allow the patient some time to work through the image so it is both elaborate and a true representative of their experience. From now on avoid talking about the pain and refer only to the image on the screen.
4. Ask the patient to sample an area with an orange/yellow—slight pain (the drop function) and apply it to a green/blue area. You want to do so until they can experience discomfort growing.
5. Only then, ask the patient to sample an area with a blue/green colour (the drop function) and apply it to a red/orange area. They can repeat it until a change is experienced.

It is helpful if the clinician assumes this process will work. If the patient is sceptic, one of the useful ways to secure cooperation is to suggest they act as if this is working, stressing that it is not important to believe in the technique in order for it to work.

16.2 Medically Unexplained Symptoms

Nicole, a twenty-six-year-old woman, sought psychotherapy following her physician's referral. She suffered from intermittent episodes of blindness—some of these episodes were partial visual impairment and others full loss of sight. All medical tests, including neurological, optical, and psychiatric, found no explanation. The 'blind' episodes were all very short, lasting only a few seconds, but were frightening and dangerous (she stopped driving and doing other activities that required focus).

At first, I was reluctant to accept Nicole as a patient. Her symptoms seemed so extreme and so medical, that I felt ill-equipped to work with her therapeutically. We agreed to meet for three sessions, and given the almost immediate improvement in her condition, I was willing to work with her, while our work was supported by her family physician.

Medically unexplained symptoms (MUS) are very common in medical practice and constitute a convoluted blend of both physical and psychological symptoms (Kroenke et al., 1993; Payne & Stott, 2010). Feasible and effective interventions applicable in medical practice have been reiterated; however, both pharmacological treatments (such as antidepressant) and psychological approaches have limited effectiveness on MUS (Edwards et al., 2010; Hong & Lee, 2008; Sumathipala et al., 2008).

Lin and Payne (2014) present their clinical experience and research in the treatment of patients with MUS. They speculate that mainstream treatments are limited in their efficacy because the majority overlook the nature of MUS as a consolidation of psychological and physical elements that result from Cartesian thinking separating physical and mental health. Therefore, they propose a three-phase therapeutic approach incorporating verbal and non-verbal techniques that facilitates connection of body and mind (encouraging patients to 'be with' their symptoms and listening to them), raises the levels of awareness to the body's language as expressed through MUS (helping patients deepening their embodied experience and letting unconscious materials to arise), and aims to find explanations for body symptoms (encouraging patients to verbalise their experiences while looking for the connection between symptoms to current life situations).

Based on these principles we believe that the foundations of managing MUS should rely on a body-mind approach which consists of taking a thoroughly biopsychosocial history; listening for possible symbolic meanings of the symptom and assessing for anxiety and depression (using previously described techniques such as tracking, bodily resonance, and other body-mind communicative skills); explaining the interaction between physiological and psychological sensations; bringing up the possibility of implicit psychological elements into explicit awareness; and recommending taking part in activities that deepen body and mind connection (such as mindfulness).

During a seemingly irrelevant conversation, which was part of my attempt to understand Nicole's support system, we talked about her boyfriend. The twenty-six-year-old woman was engaged to her boyfriend of fourteen years (since they were twelve years old). As she was describing the upcoming wedding, which was planned for the summer, Nicole suddenly experienced a loss of sight.

After the initial surprise, and thanks to Nicole's open exploration, we discovered that she was doubting the relationship with her fiancé yet felt unable to fully acknowledge it, since they had been together for so long. We spent three further months talking about her decisions and hopes, and her symptoms no longer appeared.

16.3 Stress Management

Mike is a sixty-year-old hypertensive veteran naval officer. Since his myocardial infarction a year ago, he has been suffering from uncontrolled hypertension and anxiety. Despite a normal medical investigation for secondary causes and proper compliance to his prescribed antihypertensive drugs, his blood pressure was high.

Living with chronic illness confronts us with several physical, psychological, and social intricacies. Psychological factors, such as depression and anxiety, are common in these patients (Charma & Paterniti, 1998; Fava et al., 2017; Kralik et al., 2001) and affect the quality of their lives. As already described and elaborated in previous chapters, stress might affect neuro-endocrine-immune functions resulting in responses mediated by neurotransmitters, pro inflammatory cytokines, and hormones. These might influence the pathogenesis of chronic illnesses such as hypertension (Fink, 2016; Grippo & Scotti, 2013; Theorell, 2012).

If our main presupposition of this book, that body and mind influence one another, is a useful working assumption, then it is possible, at least to some extent, to influence some of our symptoms.

After trying various pharmacological interventions with unsatisfactory out-comes, I suggested Mike practicing breathing exercises (see chapter 5) and relaxation exercises. After exercising together in the clinic while blood pres-sure is gradually returning to normal; he began practicing these exercises on a regular basis with quite beneficent outcome.

People with high blood pressure often seek tools to help them relax, let go, slow down. Teaching someone how to relax is very different than telling someone to do so.

Progressive muscle relaxation is a well-known technique of learning how to relax. Some small studies have demonstrated positive impact on somatic symptoms and chronic conditions (Lahmann et al., 2009; Loew et al., 1996). This technique is relatively time consuming, and we therefore recommend going through it with the patient once or twice and then teaching them how to use it at home. We offer here two variations of this technique, which is in var-ied use in many therapeutic modalities—from yoga, through stress manage-ment, to hypnosis and guided visualisation, and expressive psychotherapies.

Active Progressive Muscle Relaxation

This version is more suited for the patient who struggles to let go, and has not experience in doing so. It involves a similar principle to the pain scale tech-nique, in 'making something worse before making it better'.

1. Ask the patient to sit or lay down comfortably, ideally (unless they feel unsafe doing so) closing their eyes.
2. Patient takes a few deep breaths, and then holds their breath in.
3. While holding the breath in, patient is asked to tense their feet.
4. After a few seconds, ask the patient to exhale and let go of the tensing of the feet.
5. Repeat the same with the calf muscles, thighs, pelvis, stomach, back, chest, shoulders, arms and hands, face and head.
6. Then hold the breath in and tense the entire body, then let go, relax and exhale.

Encourage patient to notice sensations of relaxation, such as tingling, changes in temperature, slowing down of breathing, and more.

Passive Progressive Muscle Relaxation

A subtler version, suited for patients who find it easier to visualise or let go.

1. Ask the patient to sit or lay down comfortably, ideally (unless they feel unsafe doing so) closing their eyes.
2. Patient takes a few deep breaths

3. Patient is asked to send their attention to their feet, imagining that these receive more oxygen; relax; and become more comfortable. This could be accompanied by slow attentive and mindful breathing.
4. After a few seconds, ask the patient to exhale and let go, thus also loosening the attention to the feet.
5. Repeat the same with the calf muscles, thighs, pelvis, stomach, back, chest, shoulders, arms and hands, face and head.
6. Finally, while breathing fully, attend the body in its entirety, relax and exhale.

Encourage patient to notice sensations of relaxation, such as tingling, changes in temperature, slowing down of breathing, and more.

16.4 Conclusion

Based on accumulating data and research regarding the connection between mind and body and the interface between them as discussed all through this book, we have tried in this chapter to introduce you with practical interventions which we believe, provide you with more therapeutic tools when facing with some of the most common challenging medical conditions. In this last part of the book we presented some of the basic tents of body psychotherapy knowledge which we hope deepen your understanding of symptoms and illness, and provide you with richer therapeutic tools. Acquaintance with the language of the body, embodied diagnostic tools, and the somatic and psychic dimensions of symptoms and diseases is paramount for a deeper and broader understanding of bodily and psychological aspects interweaving in a variety of medical conditions.

References

Astin, J. (2004). Mind-body therapies for the management of pain. *Clinical Journal of Pain, 20*(1), 27–31.

Barnett, K., Mercer, S.W., Norbury, M., Watt, G., Wyke, S., & Guthrie, B. (2012). Epidemiology of multimorbidity and implications for health care, research, and medical education: A cross-sectional study. *Lancet, 380*(9836), 37–43.

Cameron, P.S.C. (2012). The need to define chronic pain self-management. *Journal of Pain Management, 5*(3), 231–236.

Charmaz, K., & Paterniti, D.A. (1998). *Health, illness, and healing: Society, social context, and self, an anthology*. Los Angeles, CA: Roxbury Publishing Company.

Edwards, M.T., Stern, A., Clarke, D.D., Ivbijaro, G., & Kasney, M.L. (2010). The treatment of patients with medically unexplained symptoms in primary care: A review of the literature. *Mental Health in Family Medicine, 7*, 209–221.

Fava, G.A., Cosci, F., & Sonino, N. (2017). Current psychosomatic practice. *Psychotherapy and Psychosomatics, 86*, 13–30.

Fink, G. (Ed.). (2016). *Stress concept and cognition, emotion, and behaviour*. San Diego, CA: Elsevier.

Gatchel, R.J., McGeary, D.D., McGeary, C.A., & Lippe, B. (2014). Interdisciplinary chronic pain management: Past, present, and future. *American Psychologist, 69*(2), 119–130.

Grippo, A.J., & Scotti, M.A. (2013). Stress and neuroinflammation. *Modern Trends in Pharmacopsychiatry, 28*, 20–32.

Hong, J.Y., & Lee, M.B. (2008). Body symptoms, pain and depression. *Journal of Taipei Medical Association, 52*, 12–14.

Kralik, D., Koch, T., & Webb, C. (2001). The domination of chronic illness research by biomedical interests. *Australian Journal of Holistic Nursing, 8*(2), 4–12.

Kroenke, K., Spitzer, R.L., Williams, J.B., Linzer, M., Hahn, S.R., DeGruy, F.V., & Broody, D. (1993). Physical symptoms in primary care: Predictors of psychiatric disorders and functional impairment. *Archives of Family Medicine, 3*, 774–779.

Lahmann, C., Witt, S., Schuster, T., Sauer, N., Ronel, J., Noll-Hussong, M., et al..(2009) Functional relaxation and hypnotherapeutic intervention as complementary therapy in asthma: A randomized, controlled clinical trial. *Psychotherapy and Psychosomatics, 78*, 233–239.

Leventhal, H. (1984). A perceptual-motor theory of emotion. In K.R. Scerer & P. Ekman (Eds.), *Approaches of emotion* (pp. 271–291). Hillsdale, NJ: Lawrence Erlbaum Associates.

Lin, Y., & Payne, H. (2014). The BodyMind Approach, medically unexplained symptoms and personal construct psychology. *Body, Movement and Dance in Psychotherapy, an International Journal for Theory, Research and Practice, 9*(3), 154–166.

Loew, T.H., Siegfried, W., Martus, P., Tritt, K., & Hahn, E.G. (1996). Functional relaxation reduces acute airway obstruction in asthmatics as effectively as inhaled Terbutaline. *Psychotherapy and Psychosomatics, 65*, 124–128.

Mäntyselkä, P.T., Turunen, J.H.O., Ahonen, R.S., & Kumpusalo, E.A. (2003). Chronic pain and poor self-rated health. *JAMA, 290*(18), 2435–2442.

McCracken, L.M., Gauntlett-Gilbert, J., & Voeles, K.E. (2007). The role of mindfulness in contextual cognitive-behavioural analysis of chronic pain-related suffering and disability. *Pain, 131*(1–2), 63–69.

McQuay, H.J.K.E., & Moore, R.A. (Eds.). (2008). *Epidemiology of chronic pain.* Seattle, WA: IASP Press.

Mills, S., Torrance, N., & Smith, B.H. (2016). Identification and management of chronic pain in primary care: A review. *Psychiatry in Primary Care, 18*(22).

Payne, H., & Stott, D. (2010). Change in the moving BodyMind: Quantitative results from a pilot study on BodyMind Approach (BMA) as groupwork for patients with Medically Unexplained Symptoms (MUS). *Counselling and Psychotherapy Research, 10*, 295–307.

Shariff, F., Carter, J., Dow, C., Polley, M., Salinas, M., & Ridge, D. (2010). Mind and body management strategies for chronic pain and rheumatoid arthritis. *Quality Health Research, 19*(8), 1037–1049.

Siegel, R.D. (2005). Psychophysiological disorders: Embracing pain. In C.K. Germer, R.D. Siegel, & P.R. Fulton (Eds.), *Mindfulness and psychotherapy* (pp. 173–196). New York, NY: Guilford Press.

Sumathipala, A., Siribaddana, S., Abeysingha, M.R.N., de Silve, P., Dewey, M., Prince, M., & Mann, A.H. (2008). Cognitive-behaviour therapy v. structured care for medically unexplained symptoms: Randomized controlled trail. *British Journal of Psychiatry, 193*(1), 51–59.

Theorell, T. (2012). Evaluating life events and chronic stressors in relation to health. *Advances in Psychosomatic Medicine, 32*, 58–71.

Torrance, N., Elliott, A.M., Lee, A.J., & Smith, B.H. (2010). Severe chronic pain is associated with increased 10 year mortality. A cohort record linkage study. *European Journal of Pain, 14*(4), 380–386.

Index

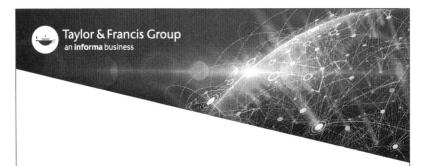